Sheryl Brahnam and Lakhmi C. Jain (Eds.)

Advanced Computational Intelligence Paradigms in Healthcare 5

Studies in Computational Intelligence, Volume 326

Editor-in-Chief
Prof. Janusz Kacprzyk
Systems Research Institute
Polish Academy of Sciences
ul. Newelska 6
01-447 Warsaw
Poland
E-mail: kacprzyk@ibspan.waw.pl

Further volumes of this series can be found on our homepage: springer.com

Vol. 302. Bijaya Ketan Panigrahi, Ajith Abraham, and Swagatam Das (Eds.)
Computational Intelligence in Power Engineering, 2010
ISBN 978-3-642-14012-9

Vol. 303. Joachim Diederich, Cengiz Gunay, and James M. Hogan
Recruitment Learning, 2010
ISBN 978-3-642-14027-3

Vol. 304. Anthony Finn and Lakhmi C. Jain (Eds.)
Innovations in Defence Support Systems 1, 2010
ISBN 978-3-642-14083-9

Vol. 305. Stefania Montani and Lakhmi C. Jain (Eds.)
Successful Case-Based Reasoning Applications-1, 2010
ISBN 978-3-642-14077-8

Vol. 306. Tru Hoang Cao
Conceptual Graphs and Fuzzy Logic, 2010
ISBN 978-3-642-14086-0

Vol. 307. Anupam Shukla, Ritu Tiwari, and Rahul Kala
Towards Hybrid and Adaptive Computing, 2010
ISBN 978-3-642-14343-4

Vol. 308. Roger Nkambou, Jacqueline Bourdeau, and Riichiro Mizoguchi (Eds.)
Advances in Intelligent Tutoring Systems, 2010
ISBN 978-3-642-14362-5

Vol. 309. Isabelle Bichindaritz, Lakhmi C. Jain, Sachin Vaidya, and Ashlesha Jain (Eds.)
Computational Intelligence in Healthcare 4, 2010
ISBN 978-3-642-14463-9

Vol. 310. Dipti Srinivasan and Lakhmi C. Jain (Eds.)
Innovations in Multi-Agent Systems and Applications – 1, 2010
ISBN 978-3-642-14434-9

Vol. 311. Juan D. Velásquez and Lakhmi C. Jain (Eds.)
Advanced Techniques in Web Intelligence 1, 2010
ISBN 978-3-642-14460-8

Vol. 312. Patricia Melin, Janusz Kacprzyk, and Witold Pedrycz (Eds.)
Soft Computing for Recognition based on Biometrics, 2010
ISBN 978-3-642-15110-1

Vol. 313. Imre J. Rudas, János Fodor, and Janusz Kacprzyk (Eds.)
Computational Intelligence in Engineering, 2010
ISBN 978-3-642-15219-1

Vol. 314. Lorenzo Magnani, Walter Carnielli, and Claudio Pizzi (Eds.)
Model-Based Reasoning in Science and Technology, 2010
ISBN 978-3-642-15222-1

Vol. 315. Mohammad Essaaidi, Michele Malgeri, and Costin Badica (Eds.)
Intelligent Distributed Computing IV, 2010
ISBN 978-3-642-15210-8

Vol. 316. Philipp Wolfrum
Information Routing, Correspondence Finding, and Object Recognition in the Brain, 2010
ISBN 978-3-642-15253-5

Vol. 317. Roger Lee (Ed.)
Computer and Information Science 2010
ISBN 978-3-642-15404-1

Vol. 318. Oscar Castillo, Janusz Kacprzyk, and Witold Pedrycz (Eds.)
Soft Computing for Intelligent Control and Mobile Robotics, 2010
ISBN 978-3-642-15533-8

Vol. 319. Takayuki Ito, Minjie Zhang, Valentin Robu, Shaheen Fatima, Tokuro Matsuo, and Hirofumi Yamaki (Eds.)
Innovations in Agent-Based Complex Automated Negotiations, 2010
ISBN 978-3-642-15611-3

Vol. 320. xxx

Vol. 321. Dimitri Plemenos and Georgios Miaoulis (Eds.)
Intelligent Computer Graphics 2010
ISBN 978-3-642-15689-2

Vol. 322. Bruno Baruque and Emilio Corchado (Eds.)
Fusion Methods for Unsupervised Learning Ensembles, 2010
ISBN 978-3-642-16204-6

Vol. 323. xxx

Vol. 324. Alessandro Soro, Vargiu Eloisa, Giuliano Armano, and Gavino Paddeu (Eds.)
Information Retrieval and Mining in Distributed Environments, 2010
ISBN 978-3-642-16088-2

Vol. 325. Quan Bai and Naoki Fukuta (Eds.)
Advances in Practical Multi-Agent Systems, 2010
ISBN 978-3-642-16097-4

Vol. 326. Sheryl Brahnam and Lakhmi C. Jain (Eds.)
Advanced Computational Intelligence Paradigms in Healthcare 5, 2010
ISBN 978-3-642-16094-3

Sheryl Brahnam and Lakhmi C. Jain (Eds.)

Advanced Computational Intelligence Paradigms in Healthcare 5

Intelligent Decision Support Systems

Springer

Dr. Sheryl Brahnam
Associate Professor
Missouri State University
Computer Information Systems
901 South National Avenue, Springfield, MO 65804, USA
E-mail: sbrahnam@missouristate.edu

Prof. Lakhmi C. Jain
Professor of Knowledge-Based Engineering
University of South Australia
Mawson Lakes Campus, South Australia, Australia
E-mail: Lakhmi.jain@unisa.edu.au

ISBN 978-3-642-26551-8 ISBN 978-3-642-16095-0 (eBook)

DOI 10.1007/978-3-642-16095-0

Studies in Computational Intelligence ISSN 1860-949X

Softcover reprint of the hardcover 1st edition 2010

Typeset & Cover Design: Scientific Publishing Services Pvt. Ltd., Chennai, India.

9 8 7 6 5 4 3 2 1

springer.com

Preface

As we enter the second decade of the 21st century, we are witnessing a radical transformation in medical care. Healthcare is becoming increasingly digital and globalized. Huge stockpiles of disparate medical information are being collected. Technologies, such as cell phones, are making unexpected headway into disease control and prevention in third world countries. Telemedicine is increasingly becoming a reality, and it is the norm now for medical diagnosis and healthcare to depend on the coordinated efforts of multiple units and teams of experts. As a result, **A**rtificial **I**ntelligence in **M**edicine (AIM) has branched out. No longer solely concerned with medical diagnosis and symbolic models of disease, or clinical encounters [1], it now embraces medical education, telemedicine, data mining, and intelligent system design.

The chapters in this volume provide the reader a glimpse of the current state of the art in intelligent support system design in the field of healthcare. We are beginning to see an outcome in the use of these systems that was once thought unlikely [2]: intelligent systems are in fact reshaping medicine and medical practice. Computer systems are doing more than simply storing, retrieving, organizing, and analyzing information [2]. As shown in the chapters in this book, these systems are changing the form as well as the substance of healthcare. They are producing new knowledge, choreographing players in complicated medical procedures, bringing top notch medical care into regions formerly lacking any care, and enabling medical practitioners to visualize, invent, and perform new procedures. These systems are also navigating the environmental challenges in healthcare as it continues to face more oversight from governmental agencies and more pressure to curtail costs.

We wish to express our gratitude to the authors and reviewers for their vision and innovative contributions. It is our privilege to introduce their work to a broader audience.

Sheryl Brahnam, USA
Lakhmi C. Jain, Australia

References

[1] Clancey, W.J., & Shortliffe, E.H. (Eds.). (1984). *Readings in medical artificial intelligence: The first decade*. Reading, MA: Addison-Wesley.
[2] Szolovits, P. (Ed.). (1982). *Artificial Intelligence and Medicine*. Boulder, CO: Westview Press.

Advanced Computational Intelligence Paradigms in Healthcare: Further Readings

[1] S. Brahnam and L.C. Jain (Editors) Advanced Computational Intelligence Paradigms in Healthcare 6: Virtual Reality in Psychotherapy, Rehabilitation, and Assessment, Springer-Verlag, 2010.

[2] S. Brahnam and L.C. Jain (Editors) Advanced Computational Intelligence Paradigms in Healthcare 5: Intelligent Decision Support Systems, Springer-Verlag, 2010.

[3] Bichindaritz, S. Vaidya, A. Jain and L.C. Jain (Editors) Advanced Computational Intelligence Paradigms in Healthcare 4: Advanced Methodologies, Springer-Verlag, 2010.

[4] M. Sardo, S. Vaidya and L.C. Jain (Editors) Advanced Computational Intelligence Paradigms in Healthcare 3, Springer-Verlag, 2008.

[5] S. Vaidya, L.C. Jain and H. Yoshida (Editors) Advanced Computational Intelligence Paradigms in Healthcare 2, Springer-Verlag, 2008.

[6] H. Yoshida, A. Jain, A. Ichalkaranje, L.C. Jain and N. Ichalkaranje (Editors) Advanced Computational Intelligence Paradigms in Healthcare 1, Springer-Verlag, 2007.

[7] N. Ichalkaranje, A. Ichalkaranje and L.C. Jain (Editors) Intelligent Paradigms for Assistive and Preventive Healthcare, Springer-Verlag, 2006.

[8] D. Husmeier, R. Dybowski and S. Roberts (Editors) Probabilistic Modelling in Bioinformatics and Medical Informatics, in Advanced Information and Knowledge Processing Series edited by L.C. Jain and X. Wu Springer-Verlag, 2005.

[9] B. Silverman, A. Jain, A. Ichalkaranje, L.C. Jain (Editors) Intelligent Paradigms in Healthcare Enterprises, Springer-Verlag, 2005.

[10] H.-N. Teodorescu and L.C. Jain (Editors) Intelligent Systems and Technologies in Rehabilitation Engineering, CRC Press, USA, 2001.

[11] A. Jain, A. Jain, S. Jain and L.C. Jain (Editors) Artificial Intelligence Techniques in Breast Cancer Diagnosis and Prognosis, World Scientific, 2000.

[12] H.-N. Teodorescu, A. Kandel and L.C. Jain (Editors) Soft Computing in Human Related Sciences, CRC Press, USA, 1999.

[13] H.-N. Teodorescu, A. Kandel and L.C. Jain (Editors) Fuzzy and Neuro-fuzzy Systems in Medicine, CRC Press, USA, 1999.

Editors

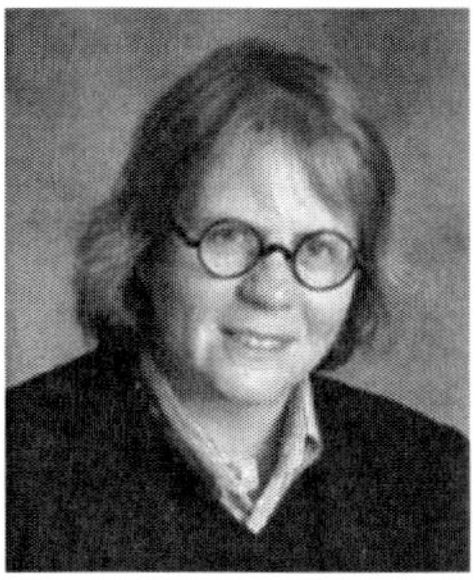

Sheryl Brahnam is the Director/Founder of Missouri State University's infant COPE (Classification Of Pain Expressions) project. Her interests focus on face recognition, face synthesis, medical decision support systems, protein descriptors, embodied conversational agents, computer abuse, and artificial intelligence. She has published a number of articles related to medicine in such journals as *Artificial Intelligence in Medicine*, *Expert Systems with Applications*, *Journal of Theoretical Biology*, *Amino Acids*, *Neural Computing and Applications*, and *Decision Support Systems*.

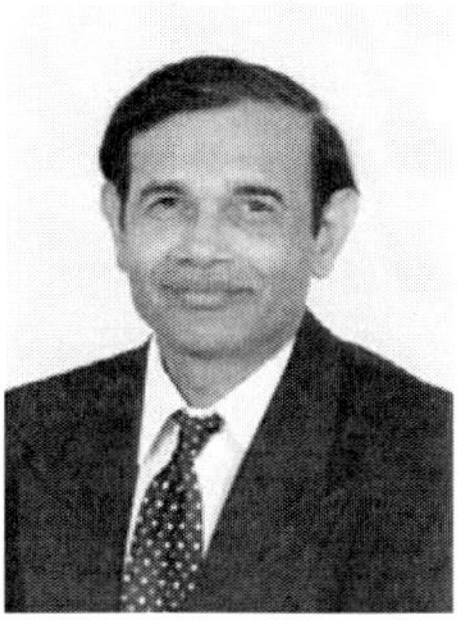

Lakhmi C. Jain is a Director/Founder of the Knowledge-based Intelligent Engineering Systems (KES) Centre, University of South Australia. He is a fellow of the Engineers Australia. He has initiated a postgraduate stream by research in the KES area. His interests focus on the applications of novel techniques such as knowledge-based systems, virtual systems, multi-agent intelligent systems, artificial neural networks, genetic algorithms, and the application of these techniques.

Contents

Part I: Clinical Decision Support Systems

Part II: Rehabilitation Decision Support Systems

Part III: Technology Acceptance in Medical Decision Support Systems

Part I

Clinical Decision Support Systems

Chapter 1
Intelligent Decision Support Systems in Healthcare

Sheryl Brahnam[1] and Lakhmi C. Jain[2]

[1] Associate Professor
Missouri State University
Computer Information Systems
901 South National Avenue,
Springfield, MO 65804, USA
sbrahnam@missouristate.edu
[2] Professor of Knowledge-based Engineering
University of South Australia
Mawson Lakes Campus,
South Australia, Australia
Lakhmi.jain@unisa.edu.au

Abstract. This chapter presents an overview of some of the most recent advances in the application of decision support systems in healthcare. A summary of the chapters on clinical decision support systems, rehabilitation decision support systems, and some current factors involving technology acceptance is presented.

1 Introduction

The field of intelligent support systems in healthcare is expanding at a rapid pace. This pace is driven by an information avalanche in health data that is unprecedented. Healthcare is incomprehensively more complex than it was at the beginning of the last century. There is no reason to believe that this complexity and the amount of new information entering the medical field will do anything more than continue to snowball. More players inside and outside of healthcare are involved in every aspect of medical care. Decision supports systems are needed if the healthcare system is successfully to navigate this turbulent environment.

The chapters presented in this volume serve as an excellent introduction to some of the opportunities being offered by the current climate. General purpose data mining techniques are being developed that can handle massive stockpiles of disparate data, and the application of decision support systems is moving into new areas, such as rehabilitation. Each of these is explored in this volume.

The chapters in this book also look hard at some of the problems being faced by the medical field. Of primary importance is the development of innovative intelligent support systems that work well with others and that can handle multiple sources of information. Medical units no longer work in isolation. They must now work together while simultaneously maintaining the autonomy needed to incorporate new

S. Brahnam & L.C. Jain (Eds.): Adv. Comput. Intell. Paradigms in Healthcare 5, SCI 326, pp. 3–10.
springerlink.com

information and the latest technologies. Systems must be developed that can orchestrate the complex work flow. Robust systems that can handle uncertainty also need to be developed.

Finally, the chapters in this book draw attention to the human element. There is the public concern for maintaining privacy while nonetheless providing information to those who need it. Governmental restrictions and policies are constantly balancing the rights and needs of its citizens when it comes to healthcare. This political element must be addressed. Decision support systems must now be flexible enough to handle changes in policy. Clinical decision support systems of the future will need to consider the constraints and uncertain relationship that will exist between technology and the regulations that govern medical data. The chapters also stress that even the best systems can fail if they do not address the needs of the medical practitioners and patients using these systems.

2 Decision Support in Healthcare

The chapters included in this book are divided into the following three parts:

Part I: Clinical Decision Support Systems
Part II: Rehabilitation Decision Support Systems
Part III: Technology Acceptance in Medical Decision Support Systems

The chapters in Part I provide an interesting selection of problems that range from decision support systems that assist health professionals in coordinating procedures across domains to a detailed description of two diagnostic support system approaches: a general-purpose diagnostic decision support system using classifier ensembles and a medical diagnostic support system that combines multiagent system theory, the holoic paradigm, swarm intelligence, and decision theory. We introduce Part I with a chapter that discusses an important desideratum for CDSS, namely, the electronic medical record (EMR). These records are at the heart of many clinical decision support systems and provide an invaluable treasure trove of information that could result in many new advances if properly mined.

In Part II, we focus on new developments in building decision support systems for rehabilitation. The three chapters in this section cover data mining approaches for predicting pregnancy rate successes, gaming for rehabilitation, and intelligent decision-support in virtual reality rehabilitation.

In Part III, we look at often neglected aspects in system design that impact the acceptance and success of decision support systems.

Below we provide a synopses of each of the ten chapters following this chapter in this book.

Part I: Clinical Decision Support Systems (CDSS)

In chapter 2, *Virtualizing Health Records in the Context of Government Regulations,* Michael Meehan focuses on the constraints that privacy standards, such as HIPAA (**H**ealth **I**nsurance **P**ortability and **A**ccountability **A**ct) enacted by the U.S.

Congress in 1996, impose on the utilization of these records. Such constraints will continue to operate as more governments exercise tighter controls over healthcare. Meehan is particularly interested in addressing how privacy standards affect the design of underlying systems that use health records. He warns that future systems will need to be designed to withstand the ever-fluctuating context of governmental regulations. To drive this point home, he describes his earlier work in virtualizing the FDA approval process in the United States so that it conformed to HIPAA standards.

In this chapter, the author also takes a brief look at the uncertain future by discussing Google Health, i.e., Google's recent development of methods for sending medical records to unrelated health care providers. Currently, Google Health is not required to conform to HIPAA since Google is not a healthcare provider. It is unknown whether HIPAA regulations will soon apply to Google Health and similar companies, such as Microsoft, or whether standards will diverge for companies that are not healthcare providers. Whichever way the wind blows, Meehan provides convincing arguments that systems need to be built that are flexible enough to handle ever changing privacy regulations.

In chapter 3, *Towards Decentralised Clinical Decision Support Systems*, Paolo Besana and Adam Barker discuss the pros and cons of using centralized versus decentralized clinical support systems. The authors argue that centralization of knowledge will increasingly become less practical as clinical information grows in size and in complexity. The authors advocate decentralizing decision support systems because this would increase system flexibility, which is critical given the rapid changes taking place in medical care. Furthermore, decentralization would enable domain experts to maintain control over their protocols and datasets. This chapter illustrates the benefits of a decentralized system using as a case study the guidelines for assessing breast cancer. Also included in this chapter is a good overview of current state of the art centralized and decentralized models, with an emphasis on the OpenKnowledge project, a highly scalable choreography-based framework that provides middleware that various services can use to interact with each other.

In chapter 4, *Data Mining Based on Intelligent Systems for Decision Support Systems in Healthcare*, Loris Nanni, Sheryl Brahnam, Alessandra Lumini, and Tonya Barrier report work on creating a general purpose diagnostic decision support system that works well on a wide variety of medical problems using multiple sources of data, including patient demographics, laboratory measurements, and features extracted from signals and images. To create such a system, the authors propose using variants of ensemble methods based on perturbing features. Included in this chapter is an overview of general methods for constructing ensembles and a more detailed tutorial on the ensemble methods, classifiers, and feature transforms and extraction methods used in the experimental section. The ensemble methods and a set of comparison stand-alone classifiers are tested using a number of benchmark medical datasets: two breast cancer datasets, a heart disease dataset, the Pima Indians dataset, a microarray dataset, and a erythemato-sequamous disease classification dataset.

In chapter 5, *Medical Diagnosis Decision Support HMAS under Uncertainty HMDSuU*, Alkaysi Esra, Rainer Unland, Weihs Claus, and Branki Cherif report their work on developing a medical diagnostic support system using multiagent system theory, the holoic paradigm, swarm intelligence, and decision theory. The focus of the chapter is on the decision process using decision theory under uncertainty, especially Baysian probability. The authors explain in detail how the HMDSuU diagnostic system is capable of finding the best diagnosis even when given scant information. The description of the HMDSuU diagnostic system is backed up by the presentation of considerable background material in decision theory, especially decision making under uncertainty. Also included in this chapter is a short description of multiagent systems, swarm intelligence, and other diagnostic and expert systems currently in use or in development.

Part II: Rehabilitation Decision Support Systems

In chapter 6, *A Data Mining Approach for Predicting the Pregnancy Rate in Human Assisted Reproduction*, Loris Nanni, Alessandra Lumini, and Claudio Manna present a clinical decision support system for deciding when the endometrium is receptive for embryo implantation. Successful pregnancy in *in vitro* fertilization (IVF)/intracytoplasmic injection (ICSI) depends on several factors: the number and quality of oocytes/embryos, uterine receptivity, and the age of the woman. Unfortunately, IVF fails in most patients. A major problem in timing ICSI is the lack of a good set of predictors related to an IVF-ICSI cycle (age of patient, endometrial and subendometrial vascularization indexes, etc.) for predicting pregnancy outcomes using IVF. The authors evaluate different feature sets in combination with various classifier ensembles with the aim of optimizing prediction accuracy and report good success using a random subspace of decision trees. This chapter provides a review of the literature on machine learning as applied to this problem. It also describes the predictors of IVF success.

In chapter 7, *Agent-Based Monitoring of Functional Rehabilitation Using Video Games*, Stuart T. Smith, Amir Talaei-Khoei, Mililani Ray, and Pradeep Ray discuss the issues involved in designing agent-based systems for rehabilitation treatments that use video games. Video games offer the advantage of allowing patients to continue working on rehabilitation tasks in a fun environment away from rehabilitation centers. The authors note that gaming for rehabilitation is more complex than what is offered by off the shelf games, which are typically too physically and cognitively challenging for rehabilitation patients. Rehabilitation games need to collect information about patient compliance and progress that could be analyzed by healthcare specialists. These games also need to incorporate the expertise and motivational capacities of rehabilitation practitioners. These as well as other possibilities offered by gaming and mobile technology are explored by the authors in a way that will encourage communication between technology and rehabilitation specialists. Included in the chapter is background information on the rehabilitation of stroke patients and those suffering spinal cord injuries, an overview of virtual reality and video gaming in healthcare practice, and a section that discusses agent-based mobile health monitoring. One contribution of the chapter is the presentation of a usability evaluation framework for evaluating mobile health monitoring in rehabilitation games played at home.

In chapter 8, *Intelligent Decision-Support in Virtual Reality Healthcare and Rehabilitation*, A. L. Brooks, who has a background both in rehabilitation and in performance art, presents a model for optimizing motivation in rehabilitation training using virtual reality. This model was developed out of the rehabilitation system known as SoundScapes that works within a Virtual Interactive Space (VIS). In VIS, profoundly disabled patients use physical movements to control game playing, painting, and music making in virtual reality environments. The open-ended system collects body function signal data as unobtrusively as possible, and the feedback mirrors user actions within virtual space using Aesthetic Resonance, which is the recognition of associations between physical action and abstract feedback. The model, called the **Z**one **O**f **O**ptimized **M**otivation (ZOOM), shows how facilitator intervention optimizes motivation and how session material can be iteratively analyzed to optimize knowledge about the patient to facilitate system adaptation to the user. As with Smith et. al., in chapter 7, Brooks sees a need for developing more intelligent rehabilitation systems. ZOOM is one step in the direction of building nontrivial decision support rehabilitation systems that are capable of empowering disabled people both by expanding their perceptions of what is possible and by employing feedback that does not necessarily engage them at the conscious level. Included in this chapter is background material on the SoundScapes system, rehabilitation motivation, and facilitator intervention. The main contribution of the chapter, is the intervention model for decision making that optimizes participant mirroring using the concept of ZOOM.

Part III: Technology Acceptance in Medical Decision Support Systems

In chapter 9, *Image-Guided Surgery and Its Adoption*, Michael Meehan discusses some of the issues related to the adoption of image-assisted surgery. While image-assisted surgery has experienced tremendous growth since the 1990s and has produced a number of benefits, including improved patient outcomes and reduced surgical time, adoption of this technology has lagged behind. In this chapter Meehan addresses some of these issues using as case studies a couple of systems he developed that were not accepted. These systems assisted surgeons in performing mandibular distraction, a procedure where bones are severed and pulled apart to facilitate growth in the bone, and craniosynostosis, where separate pieces of skull bone are reshaped on the child's head to correct for prematurely formed sutures. Both systems allowed surgeons to plan, practice, and model results on a virtual model of the patient generated from CT data. The systems also estimated how the patient would look after the procedures. The software ran on ordinary PCs with a few specific memory and graphic card requirements. The benefits offered by these systems were considerable and included reduced morbidity and mortality, reduced cost, and better outcomes. Yet they were not accepted. In contrast to these systems, the chapter discusses medical technology that has been successfully adopted, for example, MRIs and Laparoscopy (which took over 200 years to be adopted). The chapter concludes by discussing problems with the adoption of new technologies in surgery, including economics, the learning curve, and the addition of stages to the procedure. He found that the introduction of new preoperative planning steps that take place outside the operating room was especially prohibitive.

In chapter 10, *The Role of Presence in Healthcare Technology Applications*, Paul Skalski addresses the role of presence, defined as "the perceptual illusion of nonmediation," as it pertains to intelligent decision support systems in healthcare. The author argues that understanding presence can help us understand why certain systems are more successful than others. This in turn can enable us to build better theories and models. Included in this chapter is a rather complete discussion of the importance of the notion of presence in virtual reality and how it can be applied more widely. This discussion also provides a quick overview of virtual reality technologies in medicine.

In chapter 11, *Witnessed Presence in Merging Realities in Healthcare Environments*, Caroline Nevejan and Frances Brazier present their framework YUTPA (being with **Y**ou in **U**nity of **T**ime, **P**lace, and **A**ction) for the design of technology environments that explicitly orchestrate and account for how individuals perceive and witness each other. In any social interaction, how individuals witness each other has social and psychological consequences. In medical systems, where patients are required to interact with a plethora of systems, rounds robots, and virtual therapeutic environments, this element cannot be avoided and thus needs addressing if trust is to be established and if the psychological wellbeing of patients is to be nurtured in their interaction with these systems. Included in this chapter is background information on the concept of witnessing, especially the philosopher Oliver's characterization of how people witness to each other in terms of response-ability, address-ability, and the performance of testimony and transparency. Also included in this chapter is a detailed discussion of the four dimensions of the YUTPA model: space, time, action and relation. The chapter concludes by presenting some ideas on how this model can be applied in the design of medical systems.

3 Conclusion

This book is a continuation of the previous volumes [1-4] of our series on *Advanced Computational Intelligence Paradigms in Healthcare*. The recent advances in computational intelligence paradigms have highlighted the need of intelligent systems in healthcare. The primary aim of this series is to report the emerging paradigms of computation intelligence and applications in healthcare.

References

[1] Yoshida, H., Jain, A., Ichalkaranje, A., Jain, L.C., Ichalkaranje, N. (eds.): Advanced Computational Intelligence Paradigms in Healthcare 1. Springer, Heidelberg (2007)
[2] Vaidya, S., Jain, L.C., Yoshida, H. (eds.): Advanced Computational Intelligence Paradigms in Healthcare 2. Springer, Heidelberg (2008)

[3] Sardo, M., Vaidya, S., Jain, L.C. (eds.): Advanced Computational Intelligence Paradigms in Healthcare 3. Springer, Heidelberg (2008)
[4] Bichindaritz, I., Vaidya, S., Jain, A., Jain, L.C. (eds.): Advanced Computational Intelligence Paradigms in Healthcare 4. Springer, Heidelberg (2010)

Further Reading

[5] Cerrito, P.B.: Choice of Antibiotic in Open Heart surgery. Intelligent Decision Technologies-An International Journal 1(1-2), 63–69 (2007)
[6] De Paz, J.F., et al.: Case-based Reasoning as a Decision Support System for Cancer Diagnosis: A Case Study. International Journal of Hybrid Intelligent Systems 6(2), 97–110 (2009)
[7] Goel, P., et al.: On the Use of Spiking Neural Networks for EEG Classification. International Journal of Knowledge-Based and Intelligent Engineering Systems 12(4), 295–304 (2008)
[8] Hüllermeier, E.: Case Based Approximate Reasoning. Springer, Heidelberg (2007)
[9] Husmeier, D., Dybowski, R., Roberts, S., Wu, X., Jain, L.C. (eds.): Probabilistic Modelling in Bioinformatics and Medical Informatics. Advanced Information and Knowledge Processing. Springer, Heidelberg (2005)
[10] Ichalkaranje, N., Ichalkaranje, A., Jain, L.C. (eds.): Intelligent Paradigms for Assistive and Preventive Healthcare. Springer, Heidelberg (2006)
[11] Jain, A., Jain, A., Jain, S., Jain, L.C. (eds.): Artificial Intelligence Techniques in Breast Cancer Diagnosis and Prognosis. World Scientific, Singapore (2000)
[12] Kabassi, K., et al.: Specifying the personalization reasoning mechanism for an intelligent medical e-learning system on Atheromatosis: An Empirical Study. Intelligent Decision Technologies-An International Journal 2(3), 179–190 (2008)
[13] Kang, E., et al.: Remote Control Multiagent System for u-Healthcare Service. In: Nguyen, N.T., Grzech, A., Howlett, R.J., Jain, L.C. (eds.) KES-AMSTA 2007. LNCS (LNAI), 4496, 636–644. Springer, Heidelberg (2007)
[14] Kodogiannis, V.S., et al.: An Intelligent Decision Support Systems for Bacterial Clinical Isolates in Vitro Utisising an Electronic Nose. Intelligent Decision Technologies-An International Journal 3(4), 219–231 (2009)
[15] Kodogiannis, V.S.: Decision Support Systems in Wireless Capsule Endoscopy. Intelligent Decision Technologies-An International Journal 1(1-2), 17–32 (2007)
[16] Koleszynska, J.: GIGISim-The Intelligent Telehealth System: Computer Aided Diabetes Management – A New Review. In: Apolloni, B., Howlett, R.J., Jain, L. (eds.) KES 2007, Part I. LNCS (LNAI), 4692, 789–796. Springer, Heidelberg (2007)
[17] Kostakis, H., et al.: A Computational Algorithm for the Risk Assessment of Developing Acute Coronary Syndromes using Online Analytical Process Methodology. International Journal of Knowledge Engineering and Soft Data Paradigms 1(1), 85–99 (2009)
[18] Koutsojannis, C., Hatzillygeroudis, I.: Fuzzy-Evolutionary Synergism in an Intelligent Medical Diagnosis System. In: Gabrys, B., Howlett, R.J., Jain, L.C. (eds.) KES 2006. LNCS (LNAI), 4252, 1313–1322. Springer, Heidelberg (2006)
[19] Mateo, R.M.A., et al.: Mobile Agent Using Data Mining for Diagnostic Sup-port in Ubiquitous Healthcare. In: Nguyen, N.T., Grzech, A., Howlett, R.J., Jain, L.C. (eds.) KES-AMSTA 2007. LNCS (LNAI), 4496, 795–804. Springer, Heidelberg (2007)

[20] Menolascina, F., et al.: Fuzzy rule Induction and Artificial Immune Systems in Female Breast cancer Familiarity Profiling. International Journal of Hybrid Intelligent Systems 5(3), 161–165 (2008)
[21] Nebot, A.: Rule-Based Assistance to Brain Tumor Diagnosis Using LR-FIR. In: Lovrek, I., Howlett, R.J., Jain, L.C. (eds.) KES 2008, Part II. LNCS (LNAI), 5178, 173–180. Springer, Heidelberg (2008)
[22] Nejad, S.G., et al.: An Agent-based Diabetic Patient Simulation. In: Nguyen, N.T., Jo, G.-S., Howlett, R.J., Jain, L.C. (eds.) KES-AMSTA 2008. LNCS (LNAI), 4953, 832–841. Springer, Heidelberg (2008)
[23] Jeong, C.-W., Kim, D.-H., Joo, S.-C.: Mobile Collaboration Framework for u-Healthcare Agent Services and its Application Using PDAs. In: Nguyen, N.T., Grzech, A., Howlett, R.J., Jain, L.C. (eds.) KES-AMSTA 2007. LNCS (LNAI), 4496, 747–756. Springer, Heidelberg (2007)
[24] Okamoto, T., Ishida, Y.: Towards an Immunity-based System for Detecting Masqueraders. International Journal of Knowledge-based and Intelligent Engineering Systems 13(3,4), 103–110 (2009)
[25] Papageorgiou, E., et al.: Combining Fuzzy Cognitive Maps with Support Vector Machines for Bladder Tumor Grading. In: Gabrys, B., Howlett, R.J., Jain, L.C. (eds.) KES 2006. LNCS (LNAI), 4251, 515–523. Springer, Heidelberg (2006)
[26] Pous, C., et al.: Diagnosing Papients with a Combination of Principal Component Analysis and Cased Based Reasoning. International Journal of Hybrid Intelligent Systems 6(2), 111–122 (2009)
[27] Qian, Y.-W., et al.: An On-line Decision Support System for Diagnosing Hematologic Malignancies by Flow Cytometry Immunophenotyping. International Journal of Medical Engineering and Informatics 1(1), 109–124
[28] Rakus-Andersson, E.: Fuzzy and Rough Techniques in Medical Diagnosis and Medication. Springer, Heidelberg (2007)
[29] Sardo, M., Vaidya, S., Jain, L.C. (eds.): Advanced Computational Intelligence Paradigms in Healthcare, 3. Springer, Heidelberg (2008)
[30] Seta, K., et al.: Learning Environment for Improving Critical Thinking Skills in Nursing Domain. International Journal of Advanced Intelligence Paradigms 1(2) (2008)
[31] Silverman, B., Jain, A., Ichalkaranje, A., Jain, L.C. (eds.): Intelligent Paradigms in Healthcare Enterprises. Springer, Heidelberg (2005)
[32] Tentori, M., et al.: Privacy-Aware Autonomous agents for Pervasive Health-care. IEEE Intelligent Systems 21(6), 55–62 (2006)
[33] Teodorescu, H.-N., Jain, L.C. (eds.): Intelligent Systems and Technologies in Rehabilitation Engineering. CRC Press, USA (2001)
[34] Teodorescu, H.-N., Kandel, A., Jain, L.C. (eds.): Fuzzy and Neuro-fuzzy Systems in Medicine. CRC Press, USA (1999)
[35] Teodorescu, H.-N., Kandel, A., Jain, L.C. (eds.): Soft Computing in Human Related Sciences. CRC Press, USA (1999)
[36] Tonfoni, G., Jain, L.C. (eds.): Innovations in Decision support Systems. Advanced Knowledge International, ch. 8, 9 (2003)
[37] Velikova, M.: A Decision support system for Breast Cancer Detection in Screening Programs. In: Proceedings of the 18th European Conference on Artificial Intelligence, 658–662. IOS Press, Amsterdam (2008)
[38] Wagholikar, K.V., Deshpande, A.W.: Fuzzy Relation Based Modeling for Medical Diagnostic Decision Support: Case Studies. International Journal of Knowledge-Based and Intelligent Engineering Systems 12(5-6), 319–326 (2008)

Chapter 2
Virtualizing Health Records in the Context of Government Regulations

Michael Meehan

Knobbe Martens Olson & Bear, 1717 Pennsylvania Ave NW, Ste 900, Washington, DC
meehan@stanfordalumni.org

Abstract. During recent years, an increasing number of health records have become virtual or electronic. This chapter discusses some of my early work in virtualization of health records in the context of the FDA drug approval process. The chapter also outlines the lesser-known area of government regulation of virtualized or electronic health records governed by HIPAA and related standards. The constraints imposed by these regulations do not impose impossible obstacles, but they do provide constraints that are as real as any other underlying system or design constraint. This chapter then continues to discuss other current systems, such as the Kaiser and veterans health association virtual health records systems, and forward-looking systems, such as Google Health, and how these systems may relate to and be constrained by the current government data standards.

Keywords: electronic health records, personal health records, health privacy, data security, HIPAA, health information privacy.

1 Overview and History of Health Records

Around 2000, in the early days of the Internet, I designed systems and architectures for virtualizing the FDA approval process, which had operated primarily in a paper-based fashion up until that point. Since that time, the government has engaged far more in the promotion and regulation of virtual health records. As for my early work, many of the technologies used at that time are now more commonly-known and understood. What is less well known and well understood, even today, is how technology and architecture choices must be made in the context of the regulations, and how those regulations provide important and real constraints on the technologies and architectures used. This paper starts with a brief overview of the long history of health records, continues with a discussion of my early work in the virtualization of health records, and then continues with a look into the future of electronic health records and the uncertain relationship between current systems and the regulations that govern the data.

S. Brahnam & L.C. Jain (Eds.): Adv. Comput. Intell. Paradigms in Healthcare 5, SCI 326, pp. 11–26.
springerlink.com

1.1 Medical Records over Time

Medical records may be as old as the pyramids. The ancient Egyptians may have been the first to use medical records. Medical records were recorded on a papyrus, which is often called the Edward Smith Surgical Papyrus after the gentleman who purchased the papyrus in 1862, are believed to have been contributed to by three doctors in the period from 3000 to 2200 BC. It is probably more accurately described as a text book, or perhaps what doctors term today as a collection of 'case studies,' because it appears to have been written for instructional purposes. It relates the conditions of particular patients in detailed text and illustrates that doctors were thinking about and adept at recording medical records for longitudinal purposes thousands of years ago.[1]

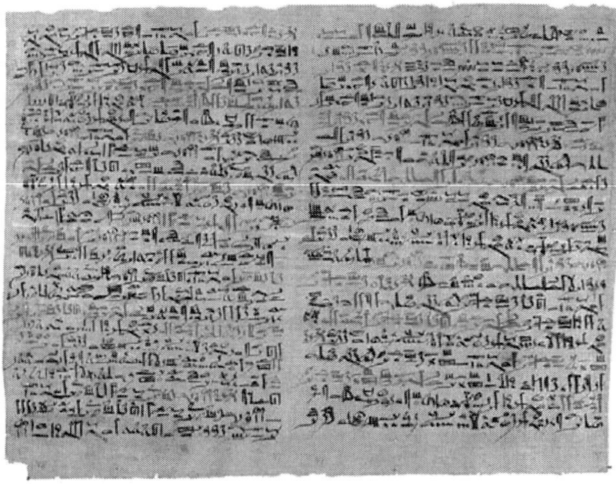

Fig. 1. The ancient Egyptian surgical papyrus known as the Edwin Smith Surgical Papyrus, evidence of medical records as long ago as 3000 BC

Over the centuries and millennia since the ancient Egyptians engaged in their pioneering medical efforts, medicine has developed, and along with it, the medical record. Certain forms of medical advances can be appreciated for both of Hippocrates' dual goals for medical records: diagnosis and record keeping.[2] In 1895, X-ray imaging was invented.[3] It allowed doctors to non-invasively silhouette bony structures inside the body. X-ray imaging resulted in great, and now ubiquitous, diagnostic advances in orthopedics and other fields relating to broken bones, structural anomalies, and joint function. The x-ray is also a medical record. X-ray film can be used to study a patient's recovery and provide a medical history for the patient. Magnetic resonance imaging (MRI), approved by the U.S. Food and Drug Administration in 1984, also serves the dual purpose of being a diagnostic device and a medical record.[4]

Not all medical records are also diagnostic. Many are written or typed notes and recollections of symptom and physiological states. Heart rate, blood pressure, and white blood cell count are often measured over time as they provide a glimpse into the state and recovery of a patient. These have traditionally been recorded on paper, and often started on the chart at the end of a patient's bed or slipped into a folder on the examination room door. Once the examination or hospital stay has been completed, the paper records are stored in a cabinet, room, or warehouse for later retrieval.

The vast number of medical records stored for possible later retrieval is daunting. Hospitals and medical providers will often have storage rooms or warehouses filled with medical records. The longitudinal nature of storing medical records can provide baselines that allow a doctor to make a diagnosis based on the individual patient's physiological changes over time. Therefore, storing medical records is critical to the medical profession.

1.2 Virtual vs. Physical Medical Records

As noted above, society is progressing in the adoption and acceptance of virtual health records. Virtualizing and electronic storage of medical records provide numerous benefits over paper records, but also raise several issues. A handful of hard drives can replace a room full of physical records. But the electronic storage of medical records brings up many specters of privacy concerns. Privacy risks are not, however, unique to electronic health records. Most of the risks that exist for medical records existed long before the virtualization of the medical records. It is in the nature of data that it is discoverable, whether that data is electronic or physical. And it is in the nature of important data that its appropriation can be an issue for those to whom the data relates, for those who are required or positioned to protect it, and for those whose industry relies on the protection of the data.

Although society is more acutely aware of the security risks of electronic medical records, physical medical records have the same inherent problems. As recently as 2008, paper medical records, instead of being destroyed, were shipped to a surplus store and sold as scrap paper. These medical records contained the social security numbers, identities, and medical history of numerous patients.[5] As another example, CVS pharmacy recently settled a suit with the government related to data privacy in which CVS had improperly discarded pill bottles and other patient information into open dumpsters.[6] As a correlate on the virtual health record side, there have been numerous reports of sensitive data being found on lost or stolen computers. For example, in 2005, a computer containing and estimated 185,000 electronic medical records was stolen.[7] In reaction to such electronic failings, the Federal Trade Commission (FTC) has issued a rule requiring companies that control electronic health records to notify customers if those electronic records have been breached or disseminated.[8]

People fear the widespread dissemination of their private information, and for good reason. The private information about illness, conditions, and well being are supremely intimate and are not the kinds of things that one would want anyone to know about without informed consent. Additionally, there is a great risk of identity theft when medical records are stolen. Medical records will typically include names, addresses, social security numbers, and financial information. Little else would be needed for a diligent thief to use existing credit or open and abuse new credit. And the identity theft may not happen immediately. The FTC's guidelines recommend, that once your identity has been stolen, to continue to monitor your credit quarterly for the first year and yearly thereafter.[9]

Although many of the risks associated with electronic health records have existed with the traditional paper and film records, it is fair to say that there are new and important risks with the virtualization of health records, and some of the existing risks have been exacerbated by the virtualization. In order to combat these risks, the U.S. government enacted the Health Insurance Portability and Accountability Act (HIPAA) and the related rules for *Security and Electronic Signature Standards*.[10,11] These two sets of rules and my early work in virtualizing clinical research are described below.

2 Clinical Research Organizations

One important arena for the virtualization of health records has been in the area of clinical research. As discussed above, this work was developed in the late 1990s and early 2000s. At the time, the technologies underlying this work were known, but not as widely used and understood as they are today. The more daunting aspect of this work was understanding and conforming with the regulatory standards that were overlaid on the technical and product requirements. This section progresses by outlining the progression of the FDA drug approval process and then discussing the architecture I developed for data protection within the context of the government regulations.

2.1 The FDA Approval and Drug-Comparison Processes

Clinical research is the process of verifying drugs for the FDA. The FDA requires a four-stage approval process for the approval of drugs. The approval process proceeds in three stages. The first phase, "Phase I" involves the side effects of a drug. These studies are usually performed on a small number of healthy volunteers, usually twenty to eighty. Based on the results and revealed toxicity and risks of the side effects identified in Phase I, Phase II will be performed. Phase II is usually an effectiveness study.

Phase II looks at those who have a certain medical condition and the effect of the drug on that condition. The tests are usually performed with at least two groups: one receiving the drug and one receiving an inactive substance or placebo. Safety and side effects continue to be monitored in this phase. The studies will typically involve three hundred or so subjects.

If there is sufficient evidence of efficacy in Phase II, then a Phase III study will be performed, usually with hundreds to thousands of patients varied over populations and ages. More information about safety and efficacy are collected, dosage is determined and drug-interactions are monitored. If the drug appears safe and effective, it gets approved by the FDA. After the drug is on the market, the pharmaceutical company must still monitored for adverse effects, safety, and effectiveness.

It is important to note that the drug approval process is handled at the individual patient level. In each phase, the drugs must be administered to an individual and the reactions of the individual must be monitored. The data from these hundreds or thousands of individuals must be collected and analyzed in order to bypass each "stage" of the FDA approval process. Traditionally, this information was collected on paper, often communicated via fax or regular mail, and the data was entered into databases in order to analyze the data mathematically to determine various aspects of the system, including the estimated sample size needed for the approval. Similar systems are used in order to show the efficacy of drugs. For example, if a company desires to run an advertisement stating that "Our drug is as effective as any other on the market," then the company would have to show that no other drug was statistically more effective than theirs is. If a company desires the ability to say that "Our drug is more effective than any comparable drug in the market," then a different level of statistical power would be needed. Specifically, the company would have to show that the drug was significantly more effective, statistically speaking. This requires both that the drug is more effective, and that enough data is collected to provide statistical significance.

In both the drug approval and drug comparison situations, collecting patient and efficacy data on paper and transmitting it via mail and fax is simultaneously inefficient and error prone. Although it may be efficient for practitioners to enter the data onto paper forms, assuming the forms are clear, well-designed, and available, the collection, retention, and data entry phases may be inefficient in numerous ways. For example, organizing thousands of individual pieces of paper containing the required data for numerous studies at a single hospital could be a very difficult task. Further, collecting and coordinating those pieces of paper over multiple hospitals is also a difficult task. Beyond that, there are inefficiencies in the transportation and storage at the collection or consolidation site.

The codification of these paper records at the collection site is potentially error prone and expensive. The person codifying the paper records may misread or misunderstand the paper records, providing one type of error. The coder may understand the record, but make a clerical error in entering the data, causing another type of error.

All of the real and possible errors and the inefficiencies have opened the way for alternatives to the paper-based approach to clinical research. In the next section, I discuss the work that I did in virtualizing the FDA approval process.

2.2 Virtualizing the FDA Approval Process

My work on the virtualization of health records in the context of government regulation lead to a particular architecture suitable for the needs of clinical research organizations. The most difficult aspect of designing the multitiered architecture was ensuring conformance with the governing standard known as HIPAA. HIPAA was enacted in 1996. In 1998 the Department of Health and Human Services proposed new rules for *Security and Electronic Signature Standards*, which apply to data stored or transmitted by healthcare providers and institutions. There is an argument that clinical research organizations are not covered under HIPAA.[12] Notwithstanding this, we decided to abide in every way possible to the HIPAA standard, and further to the data transmission and storage standards promulgated by the U.S. Department of Health and Human Services. In addition to HIPAA conformance, developing the system for virtualizing clinical research, I had to consider technical constraints and process constraints. The resulting architecture and its relation to government regulations are detailed below.

Data Collection

In many cases, especially for Phase III trials, clinical data is collected by numerous doctors and other practitioners in offices and hospitals across a wide geographic range. Data collection at these sites can happen in a number of ways. As will become apparent when looking at the system as a whole, one of the keys to data collection is collecting the data in a manner that will allow it to be electronic before the data is moved to the next state of processing or transportation. One of the obvious ways to enable electronic data collection is to have the practitioners input the data into a computer. This computer could be a desktop, laptop, or, perhaps a device that is more portable, like a personal data assistant, an ultraportable computer, etc.

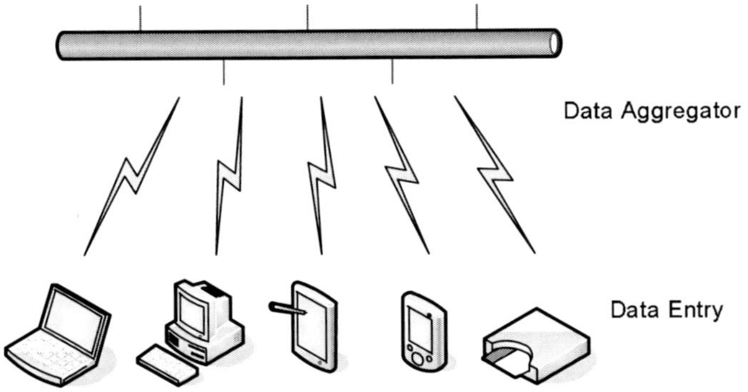

Fig. 2. Data collection of virtualized clinical trial records needs to be agnostic to data entry mechanism

These days, the issue of electronic data collection seems simple enough on its face. There are, of course, several complications. Entering patient data is only one aspect of a practitioner's otherwise busy, complicated, and important job. In many cases, patients will be separated into multiple rooms in a hospital or office.

Therefore, the data collection mechanism must be portable. As such, a desktop is likely ruled out, except in instances where data will be collected in a single room for multiple patients. A laptop would be more reasonable in most cases, but might still be awkward for transportation and data entry. Tablets and PDAs are more portable and would more easily allow movement from room-to-room as data is being entered. Another possible data entry system would be via voice. There is surely not a single solution to the data entry issue. It is clear, however, that the solution should be flexible enough to allow for multiple entry types. This is depicted in Figure 2. The data entry mechanism becomes more important as we look at other aspects of data entry, as discussed below.

Table 1. Technical Security Mechanisms to Guard Against Unauthorized Access to Data That Is Transmitted over a Communications Network, from *Security and Electronic Signature Standards*; Proposed Rule, Federal Register, Vol. 63, No. 155, (August 12, 1998), 43, 254-5

Requirement	Implementation
Communications/network controls If communications or networking is employed, the following implementation features must be implemented: Integrity controls, Message authentication. In addition, one of the following implementation features must be implemented: Access controls, Encryption. In addition, if using a network, the following four implementation features must be implemented: Alarm, Audit trail, Entity authentication, Event reporting.	Access controls. Alarm. Audit trail. Encryption. Entity authentication. Event reporting. Integrity controls. Message authentication.

This structure, of course, causes issues of data privacy. The connection of these various data entry mechanisms to a centralized network or server that will collect and consolidate the data can be wired or wireless, over an inherently encrypted connection (e.g., HTTPS, SSL, etc.), or unencrypted (e.g., FTP). Therefore, in designing the systems and the data entry for these systems, one must decide the type of data connection to be used. The Department of Health and Human Services' *Security and Electronic Signature Standards* includes a section discussing to the technical security mechanisms necessary to guard against unauthorized access to data that is transmitted over a communications network.[13] A copy of the table summarizing the technical security requirements for transmission of data is presented in Table 1.

Table 2. Technical Security Services to Guard Data Integrity, Confidentiality, and Availability, from *Security and Electronic Signature Standards*; Proposed Rule, Federal Register, Vol. 63, No. 155, (August 12, 1998), 43,254

Requirement	Implementation
Access control The following implementation feature must be implemented: Procedure for emergency access. In addition, at least one of the following three implementation features must be implemented: Context-based access, Role-based access, User-based access. The use of Encryption is optional.	Context-based access. Encryption. Procedure for emergency access. Role-based access. User-based access.
Audit controls	
Authorization control (At least one of the listed implementation features must be implemented).	Role-based access. User-based access.
Data Authentication	
Entity authentication (The following implementation features must be implemented: Automatic logoff, Unique user identification. In addition, at least one of the other listed implementation features must be implemented).	Automatic logoff. Biometric. Password. PIN. Telephone callback. Token. Unique user identification.

It appears that the standards would require encryption from the point of sending data to the point of receipt. This can be handled in a number of ways. The example most commonly known to people these days would be public key encryption. With encryption, data is collected, usually in a readable form, by the encrypting entity. In this case the encrypting entity would be the PDA, computer, or other device used to collect patient data. Without going into great detail about encryption and the various methods of encryption, we can generally say that a cipher, which is a string of letters or numbers, is used to transform and recode the readable data into an unreadable string. Only those with the key, which corresponds to the cipher, will be able to decrypt the data that has been encrypted. As with any security measure, there are possibilities that the encrypted data can be decrypted using a brute force or other algorithm for guessing the key and decrypting the data. This possibility aside, end-to-end encryption will stop 'snooping' of the data between the point of encryption, where the patient's data was first entered into the system, and the point of decryption, the central server.

The *Security and Electronic Signature Standards* also governs data storage.[14] Therefore, one must also consider the potential for temporary or transient local storage of data, and security surrounding that. The standards appear to be directed to regulating long-term storage. It is not clear, however, whether temporary or transient storage is governed by the standards. Table 2 is a reproduction of the table summarizing the data storage regulations.

It would not appear that the temporary storage of data would need access control, audit control, or any of the other aspects of the technical security defined in standards. It may suffice to ensure that the temporary data is not improperly accessible and that it is deleted or expunged within some predetermined time limit.

As a more concrete example from my work, consider a particular instance of the architecture in which a PC is running a standard Internet browser that is used to collect teaching data for clinical research. The system, as it was designed, and as used in conformance with standards, allows a doctor to input clinical data on a webpage and uploaded that data over the network to a central aggregator, as depicted in Figure 2. The connection between the personal computer, via the webpage and the central aggregator might be over an HTTPS connection. Using this architecture, data is encrypted from the time it is entered at the webpage until it is received at the aggregator. This conforms to the data security standards. In order to ensure that it also conforms to storage standards, the system simply avoids storing the webpage or any of the data from the webpage beyond the time of transmission.

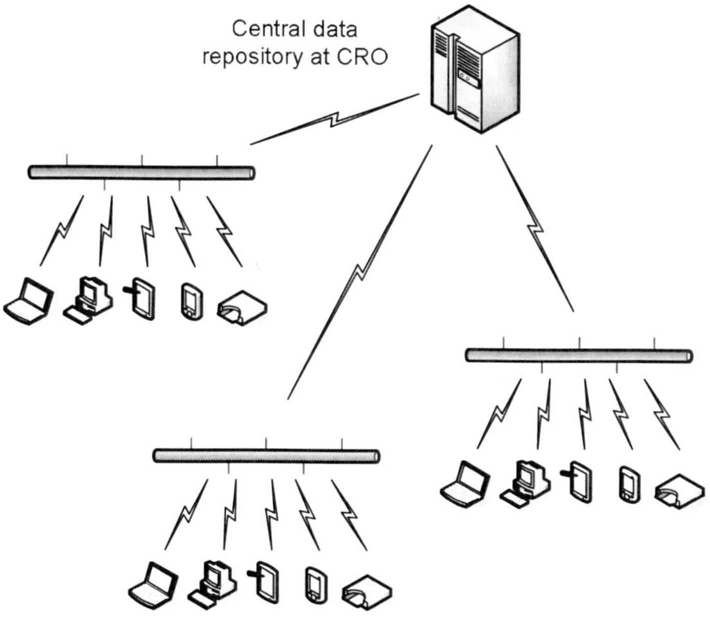

Fig. 3. Data collected at multiple research sites will be aggregated and sent to the CRO or central repository

Once the data is at the aggregator, however, we must again think about conforming to the standards. If the data at the aggregator is merely received over HTTPS, then it will be decrypted by the Web server and will exist on the aggregator as unencrypted data. Therefore, care must be taken with the data at this intermediate stage. One solution is for the system to store the data immediately into a database. Once the patient data is received as part of a web transaction over HTTPS, that data should not be stored in the web log or in any other manner. Storing the data received in a database will provide the necessary security for the data storage standard. Most modern databases will allow data to be encrypted within the database. Therefore, a malicious attacker would not be able to access the data and read it without deciphering the key to the encryption. Modern databases will also provide access control to data, auditing of the access of data, and the other security functions required by the standards.

Once data is sent from the aggregator to the central server or clinical research organization, as depicted in Figure 3, care must again be taken in the transmission and storage of the data. This is handled in a manner similar to that discussed for the transmission of data between the practitioner and the aggregator. In the system, data is extracted from the database and sent to the clinical research organization at regular intervals or as needed. For example, data will often be sent automatically in the middle of the night, when network traffic is low and data has been entered for the day.

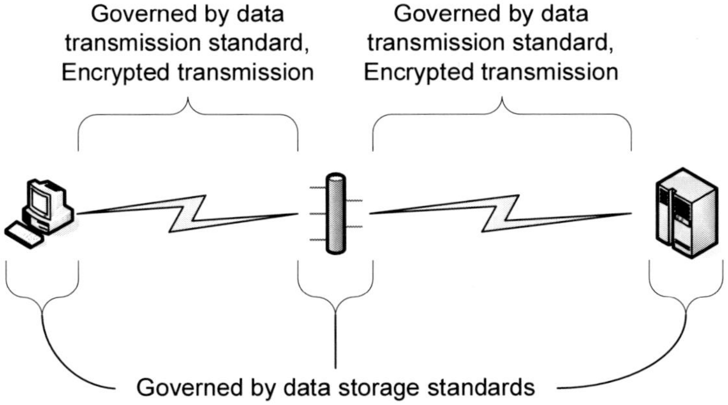

Fig. 4. Depiction of patient data and the governing standards from entry to the central server

In order to send the data, it is extracted from the database and temporarily, locally stored. This can be performed by a person or an automated process, each of which would be required to have proper access credentials, such as a username and password. Once the data is temporarily, and locally stored, it is ready to be sent to the central server. Sending the data to the central server requires the same kind of secure connection that was used in the previous transmission step. HTTPS could again be used, but a more common way for two programs to communicate would be through an SSL connection. There are important differences between these two, but in the context of this discussion, it is important to note that they both encrypt data, and do not allow it to be viewed while the data is in transmission over a network.

Given that the transmission over the network is secure, we must again turn to the storage and handling of the data. It is of course imperative that the decrypted, locally stored data at the aggregator is deleted after it has been sent. The data, upon arrival, will be decrypted and stored again in a database at the central server. As noted above, most modern databases will provide the security necessary for the government standards. A depiction of the data transfer from end-to-end is depicted in Figure 4.

Another way to comply with the standards is to use end-to-end encryption. In the end-to-end encryption, patient data would be encrypted at the source, where it was first entered, and not be decrypted until it is received at the other end. Using the same architecture as described above, this would mean that the data at the personal computer would be encrypted upon receipt. Therefore, it would be best to use something other than a webpage to collect data. The data would be instead collected in a computer program which would immediately encrypt the patient data. Encrypted patient data would then be sent to the aggregator over the network. Because the data has been encrypted, it would not necessarily have to be encrypted again over the data transmission. Further, the data would already be encrypted upon receipt of aggregator and the central server. As such, the database or other storage mechanism at the aggregator and central server would not necessarily have to encrypt the locally stored data. Once encrypted patient data is received at the central server, the central server could use the corresponding key in order to decrypt the data. This is depicted in Figure 5.

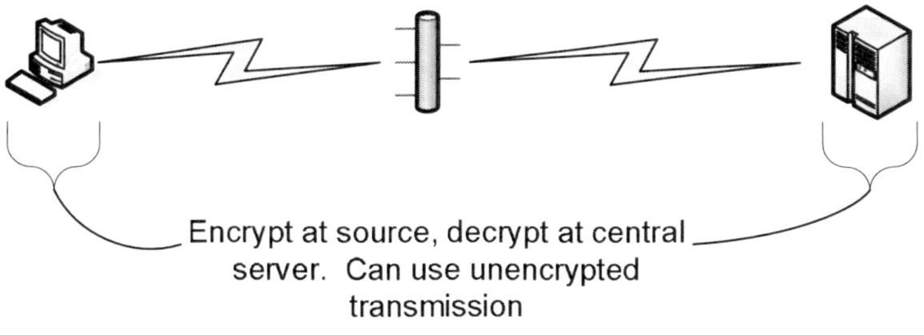

Fig. 5. Depiction of an end-to-end system for use by clinical research organizations

This architecture would provide a fairly secure transmission environment, but would have technical complications not associated with the architecture of Figure 4. Each individual data entry point would have to be able to encrypt data in a way that could be decrypted by the central server. One option for this would be for each data entry point to have the same cipher to encrypt the data, and then the central server would have a single key to decrypt all of the received data. This option would comply with the government standards, but if the single key known to the server were discovered, then all of the data associated with the patients could be decrypted. This may be too much of a security risk for some. Another downside of this architecture is that all of the data entry points would have to have the ability to encrypt the data. Most data entry devices, even PDAs, have computing capacity to encrypt data. It would require, however, that in addition to computing power, each data entry device would also have software that would encrypt the data. The problem with this is distribution – both of the original software and updates. Providing software that would run on all of the variety of data entry devices and all of the possible operating systems would be a tremendous burden on the software designers and would be prone to failure on individual data entry devices. It is this latter reason that provides the greatest deterrent to adopting this architecture.

Looking more closely at what is required for compliance with the government standards for data storage, we see that many of the requirements must be met by the central server. Access control, which would be required of the central server due to its storage of the patient data, is a feature that is commonly provided by database systems. This makes databases an obvious choice for data storage in the central server.

Looking at access control in more detail, the two most common types of access control are context-based access control and user-based access control. In context-based access control, typically, different types of user profiles or contexts are established and users are associated with those contexts. For a clinical research organization, an example access control context might be a "data analyst." A data analyst may be able to access data by patient identification number, access test results, and access dosage and treatment information. Data analysts may not be allowed to access patient identifying information, however. Another example access control context might be what is commonly called a "Superuser". A superuser may be able to access all of the information associated with the patient, including identifying information.

One of the other requirements of a government standards is audit control. The requirements for audit controls are not discussed extensively in the government standards but the standards do state that audit data should be recorded in order to "identify suspect data access activities, assess its security program, and respond to potential weaknesses." It also states that there should be "audit control mechanisms to record and examine activity."[15] Therefore, the simplest way to abide by this requirement is to record the access and manipulation activities of each user. In the context of the role-based access control system, this means that each time a user logs in with a personally-identifying user name and password, the activities performed by the user, which will be within the role-based context, are recorded and stored to a log. Of course the data accessed in-and-of-itself is not recorded, but only the actions taken by the user, such as the data analyst. With this, it should be relatively easy to determine what actions were taken by which users, which is one of the fundamental principles of the access control required by the government standards. From this data, the organization would be able to identify suspect data access activities and respond to potential weaknesses, as required by the standards.

The government standards also require physical safeguards for the data. Notably, one of these safeguards is controlling physical access to locations that store patient data. Because the patient is not stored on the data entry devices discussed above, these standards are not applicable for those devices. Patient data is stored, however, at the aggregator and the central server. Therefore, the system must be set up physically to limit access to the aggregator and to the central server. Limiting access typically will not be a problem for the central server because it will be housed either in a co-location facility that has physical security, or at the clinical research organization, which likewise has physical security. The point of greatest potential weakness is the aggregator. The aggregator will be, as discussed above, a physical computer that will typically be located geographically near or at a hospital or doctor's office. In order to abide by these standards, access to the central server will have to be physically controlled. This will typically mean placing the aggregator computer in a room that is accessible only via key card access. Because this is a standard that applies to the storage of all patient data, it should not be a problem to find such a room in a doctor's office or hospital. If this room is not available, however, a local co-location facility may be used to house the aggregator in order to protect the data stored at the aggregator.

The effect of the regulations on the development of a clinical research data aggregation system was considered above. Virtualization of health records has expanded, however, and will continue to expand. Below is a discussion of some of the existing virtual health record systems as well as systems that are poised to be the future of virtual health records.

2.3 The Current and Future Virtualization of Health Records

It is not surprising, given the growth of the Internet and the increasing comfort of the population with performing vital actions online, such as banking and purchases, that the virtualization of health records has also increased in acceptance and popularity. The veterans hospital administration (VHA) has been using electronic health records for more than a decade. Almost all of the records that they keep are electronic. A recent study has also found that approximately 1.5% of US hospitals, excluding the VHA hospitals, have a comprehensive electronic health record system.[16] All of Kaiser Permanente's ("Kaiser") clinics and hospitals operate with electronic health records.[17] These hospitals are governed by the same government data standards discussed above. That is, they are required to control access, both physically and electronically, to stored data. They are also required to audit access to the data. Any transmission of the data over a wired or wireless network must be encrypted.

The virtualization of health records has gone beyond healthcare providers such as the VHA and Kaiser to technology companies. Both Google and Microsoft now provide technologies for storing electronic health records. Here, I concentrate on the Google software, which is called Google Health. Google Health provides a central repository for electronic health records. Their basic model relies on something that does not exist, for example, for the VHA. That is, the Google Health model relies on the necessity of transferring health records among unrelated health care providers. Imagine that you move from Irvine, California to Cleveland, Ohio. If you have been treated at Hoag Hospital in Irvine before you moved, then you would have to have all of your medical records transferred to a local health care provider, such as the Cleveland Clinic. With physical medical records, which is still by far the most common, this would mean taking all your original x-rays and paper medical records and having them copied or having the originals sent to the Cleveland Clinic. If both sides have electronic medical records, then you will be able to have the Hoag Hospital transmit the electronic medical records to the Cleveland Clinic. That sounds simple enough, and it would be, if the two hospitals have compatible electronic medical records systems. As is commonly the case for electronic systems, however, this is unlikely. Therefore, even if both of the hospitals have electronic records systems, it is very likely that the two systems cannot "talk" to each other, in the electronic data sense. Therefore, the data from one hospital would have to be translated into a format that could be understood by the second hospital. This is where Google Health may help. In addition to the other services provided by Google Health, it provides interfaces to common electronic medical records systems. Google Health then stores the electronic medical records in canonical Google format. When the patient wishes to have the data sent to another hospital, the data is exported from Google and translated into the format needed by the destination hospital. As such, the patient is able to affect the transfer of electronic medical records from one hospital to another.

In addition to the translation and transmittal of electronic medical records, Google Health provides a number of other services. For example, the Cleveland Clinic operates with Google Health to provide "MyConsult," which is an online service that allows "anyone, anywhere" to have access to Cleveland Clinic physicians. The Cleveland Clinic will provide second opinions and pre-adoption and nutrition consultations via this portal.[18] There are also a number of other portals available for screening and locating sellers of prescription drugs.[19]

Although Google must comply with government rules, such as the FTC breach-reporting rule discussed above, Google Health is not covered by the government standards. The standards require only that healthcare providers and companies providing services for healthcare providers obey data standards.[20] It seems fairly well-established that Google is not covered by the standards as they are currently written. This may change over time as Google Health and Microsoft Health Vault become more widely used, and are used for a broader range of patient activity. For now, however, Google and Microsoft are not strictly required to obey the government's standards. That is not to say that the will not make every effort to protect patient data, or that they are not required to maintain privacy of their users under some other contractor requirements, but they are not required to comply with the health care related data standards. Some of the main issues of concern for this are in the transmission, storage, and sharing of personal health information. When users first login to Google Health's website they are required to click the Google Terms of Service and Sharing Authorization Agreement, which state that Google is not a covered entity under HIPAA. Google also has its own Sharing Policy and Privacy Policy, by which its users and Google are bound.

From these statements and policies, it does not appear that Google is attempting to do anything nefarious by adopting separate policies, but it is important to read them, as they differ from the government standards. Further, as Google's policies and the parallel government regulations will change over time, the two may become more divergent.

As an example of how the Google Sharing Authorization Agreement differs from how one might expect data to be shared, consider that Google Health only allows a user to share her entire profile with an provider, such as a doctor.[21] Therefore, the user will be sharing all of the data in the profile with a doctor. If she is keeping other information in her Google Health profile, such as running logs, eating habits, etc., she may not want to share all the information with the doctor. It does appear that Google Health will allow you to create more than one profile, however. Therefore, a user can create one profile to share with her doctor, and another one in which more information is stored. Creating multiple profiles seems counterintuitive, and the purpose for it is only apparent if you read the Google Health Sharing Authorization Agreement. Further, directly contrary to government regulations for hospitals, Google will share a user's health information in limited instances. Google's Privacy Policy states that Google will share information in order to avoid fraud to satisfy laws, or to "protect against harm to the rights, property or safety of Google, its users or the public as required or permitted by law."[22] HIPAA would not appear to give organizations such broad leeway in disclosing electronic health records of the patient. Google may never act on this provision in its Privacy Policy with respect to health records, but it is important for users to know that this disclosure provision exists in Google's Privacy Policy, in contrast to standards in parallel government regulations.

3 Conclusion

The way we handle, think, about, and regulate health records has gone through transitions over time, and will continue to change. Those who design systems for handling virtual health records must be aware of not only the technical and design requirements, but also the regulations that govern those systems. Currently, the entities covered under HIPAA are limited, but as more and more technology companies get involved in virtualizing health records, the regulations may change and may be expanded to cover a broader range of entities in the virtual health record sphere.

References

1. Finger, S.: Origins of neuroscience: a history of explorations into brain function, pp. 6–8. Oxford University Press, Oxford (2001)
2. National Institutes of Health, National Center for Research Resources, Electronic Health Records Overview (April 2006)
3. Peters, P., Roentgen, W.C., the discovery of X-rays: Textbook of Radiology, http://www.medcyclopaedia.com/library/radiology

4. McGivney, W.T.: Approval Processes Different for Devices and Drugs. Physician Executive (July 1990)
5. Medical records sold to teacher as scrap paper, Associate Press (March 10, 2008), http://www.msnbc.msn.com/id/23561667
6. CVS Caremark Settles FTC Charges, Failed to Protect Medical and Financial Privacy of Customers and Employees, Also Pays $2.25 Million to Settle Allegations of HIPAA Violations (February 18, 2009), http://www.ftc.gov/opa/2009/02/cvs.shtm
7. Kawamoto, D., Medical group: Data on 185,000 people was stolen, ZD Net (April 8, 2005)
8. FTC Issues Final Breach Notification Rule for Electronic Health Information (August 17, 2009), http://www.ftc.gov/opa/2009/08/hbn.shtm
9. Federal Trade Commission, About Identity Theft, http://www.ftc.gov/bcp/edu/microsites/idtheft/consumers/about-identity-theft.html
10. U.S. Department of Health and Human Services, Summary of the HIPAA Privacy Rule, http://www.hhs.gov/ocr/privacy/hipaa/understanding/summary/privacysummary.pdf
11. Security and Electronic Signature Standards; Proposed Rule, Federal Register, vol. 63(155) (August 12, 1998).
12. Association of Clinical Research Organizations, Guidance Clarifies Impact of Privacy Rule on Researchers and CROs (December 2002)
13. Supra note 10 at pp. 43254 – 43255
14. Supra note 10
15. Supra note 10at p. 43254
16. Jha, A., et al.: Use of Electronic Health Records in U.S. Hospitals. New England Journal Of Medicine 360, 1628, 1631 (2009)
17. Kaiser Permanente Completes Electronic Health Record Implementation (March 3, 2010), http://xnet.kp.org/newscenter/pressreleases/nat/2010/030310ehrcomplete.html
18. Google Health Partner Profile, Cleveland Clinic (2009), http://static.googleusercontent.com/external_content/untrusted_dlcp/www.google.com/en/us/intl/en-US/health/about/partners/Cleveland_Clinic.pdf
19. Google Health, Personal Health Services, https://health.google.com/health/directory?cat=importrecords
20. Supra note 13 at p. 43244
21. Google Health Sharing Authorization (April 28, 2008), http://www.google.com/intl/en-US/health/sharingauth.html
22. Google Privacy Policy (March 11, 2009), http://www.google.com/privacypolicy.html

Chapter 3
Towards Decentralised Clinical Decision Support Systems

Paolo Besana[1] and Adam Barker[2]

[1] Universite de Rennes, France
[2] University of St Andrews, United Kingdom

Abstract. The sheer quantity and complexity of medical information, even within a single speciality, is beyond the power of one person to comprehend. Clinical decision support (CDS) systems have been clearly demonstrated to improve practice by removing complexity and aiding the decision making process for clinicians. However, the specific pieces of information most relevant to a particular clinical decision are typically scattered over a wide range of databases, applications, journals and written notes. Centralisation of knowledge is becoming less practical as the volume and complexity of data increases. Through a motivating scenario taken from the field of cancer research, we argue against complete centralisation and towards an open, decentralised architecture, allowing domain experts to curate and maintain their own processes and data sets. We introduce the UK-based Safe and Sound project and propose an architecture based on PRO*forma*, a formal language for describing CDS systems and OpenKnowledge, an enabling technology for decentralised agent-based systems. We demonstrate that although more complex to initially model, our architecture scales with increasing complexity, is more flexible and reliable than architectures which rely on centralisation.

Keywords: Clinical decision support systems, medical guidelines, workflow, service choreography.

1 Introduction

Many science-based fields are facing a knowledge crisis, in that knowledge is expanding while economic resources and the human capacity to apply it remain finite. Medicine is perhaps the most prominent example; the field is the focus of a vast and productive research effort, but new tools and techniques are not always either quickly disseminated or effectively used. In the last thirty years, clinicians and computer scientists have developed technologies that could hold the key to managing that ever-growing complexity. Research on computerised Clinical Decision Support (CDS), Workflow and Knowledge Management systems has blossomed into a global movement, with applications in most areas of medicine.

Although healthcare brings enormous benefits to us all, there is compelling evidence that avoidable errors are common and patients are frequently harmed. Medical guidelines synthesise the latest evidence and best practice for a particular clinical

S. Brahnam & L.C. Jain (Eds.): Adv. Comput. Intell. Paradigms in Healthcare 5, SCI 326, pp. 27–44.
springerlink.com

condition or intervention. They are produced and used in many countries and have been shown to significantly improve healthcare outcomes [16]. CDS systems apply formalised (computer-interpretable) medical knowledge to patient data in order to arrive at patient-specific treatment recommendations and guidelines in a way that ensures best practice.

The evidence [18] that these technologies can have the desired effects (improving clinician performance, patient outcomes, and the cost-effectiveness of health centres, among others) is substantial, but at present no one knows how to deploy these systems in a safe, sound, and scalable way. A major challenge is how to integrate and deliver support for a variety of such services at the point of care, in the complex, unpredictable and ever-changing context of healthcare delivery, and how to do this in a flexible yet scalable and safe way.

In order to integrate software and data, academia and industry have gravitated towards service-oriented architectures. Service-oriented architectures are an architectural paradigm for building software applications from a number of loosely coupled distributed services.

Service oriented architectures are part of a wide family of middleware systems: every component exposes services accessible through the network. Complex systems can be pulled together, invoking services belonging to different and possibly external systems using workflow languages [4] like the Business Process Execution Language (BPEL) [2] or Yet Another Workflow Language (YAWL) [35]. These frameworks are based on a centralised, imperative paradigm: a central process controls everything, the other services are passive, unaware of being part of a larger, more complex workflow. In this approach, called *orchestration*, services are usually wired together into an application at design time, leaving little margin if, for example, one of the services is unavailable at run-time.

We claim that this approach does not scale well with the growing complexity of systems. This is the case, as we will see in the next sections, for medical procedures, where complex workflows, developed by committees, involve the interaction of many different actors such as desktop applications, web services, databases, diagnostic devices and monitoring tools and have to be adapted to the contingent and varying realities of hospitals and clinics. We advocate a different paradigm, based on *sharing choreographies* among actors. We believe that both design and execution of complex systems can benefit from this approach. At design-time, the choreography paradigm forces the developers to think in terms of the actors, their roles and their interactions, making them explicit and abstracting away from the details of their specific activities. While the general approach is to share description of services, and pull them together at design-time into a specific application, our approach takes the opposite direction and shares the choreographies. At execution-time, shared choreographies are the contracts that actors can search, verify and agree to follow: the binding with actors takes place at run-time, not at design-time.

The OpenKnowledge[1] project has allowed us to develop a distributed, open, peer-to-peer framework, focussed on shared interaction models that are executed by peers. In this paper we focus on the application of this framework to the

[1] `http://www.openk.org/`

coordination of medical guidelines, using as a case study the assessment procedure (called triple assessment) followed by a patient suspected of breast cancer.

This Chapter discusses the work of the UK-based Safe and Sound project[2] for eliciting grand challenges in ICT-driven healthcare and is structured as follows. In Section 2 we introduce the problem requirements of formalising and enacting medical guidelines, exemplified by the breast cancer assessment case study in Section 3. Then in Section 4 we discuss the advantages of a choreography-based approach to the problem, against an orchestration-based one. In Section 5.2 we cover OpenKnowledge, as a flexible, choreography-based framework that can address some of the requirements of medical guidelines. Related work is discussed in Section 6 and conclusions are presented in Section 7.

2 Medical Guidelines

Gaps between medical theory and clinical practice are consistently found in health service research. Care procedures can differ significantly between different health centres, with varying outcomes for patients, and medical errors could be avoided if standard procedures were followed consistently. One of the causes of discrepancies in care is the difficulty in distributing and sharing efficiently the large volume of information continuously produced by medical research. These issues have pushed the development of clinical practice guidelines: several studies [21] have shown that published guidelines can improve the quality of care.

Guidelines are usually defined by a committee of experts and are provided as booklets, often hundreds of pages long, covering relatively narrow fields or specific pathologies. Hundreds of guidelines are available, and generalist doctors are expected to be aware of, and follow, the guidelines relevant to each patient. The result is that guidelines are rarely followed, and inconsistencies in medical treatments are not reduced as much as hoped.

Information technology can improve the situation. Many clinical guidelines provide informal descriptions of workflows and rules that can be translated into formal, machine-executable, representations. Research has suggested that computerised clinical supports can improve practitioner compliance with guidelines [19].

Guidelines encode at least two separate types of knowledge: they specify the overall coordination between actors, both clinical and non-clinical (for example, the results of all the exams are sent to a multidisciplinary team for discussion and to the Electronic Health Record of the patient) and specific medical knowledge required in taking decisions (for example, dosing drugs or classifying a melanoma). Guidelines are developed for general adoption: the coordination specifications need to be adapted to the contingent realities of different institutions and clinics, and the medical knowledge need to be kept updated.

Finally, different guidelines specify medical procedures at different level of abstraction, from the general framework defining the milestones of screening, intervention and follow-up within the national health system, to the detail of the dosing of a specific drug. Depending on the condition and on the abstraction level, there can

[2] `http://www.clinicalfutures.org.uk/`

be varying degrees of freedom in the selection of the guideline, or in the selection of participating clinicians. For example, a woman can choose among several paths of care for her pregnancy, while the (more critical) procedure for a heart attack is more stringent. In order to enact the full pathway a patient has to go through the various specifications that should be integrated, selecting at each step the best one, and adapting them to the contingencies.

In the work described in this Chapter we use OpenKnowledge, a technology developed for distributed peer-to-peer systems, to represent, integrate and enact the coordination aspect of guidelines offering a level of flexibility that improves portability between different institutions.

Before the details of OpenKnowledge are discussed, we first introduce our case study and discuss the differences between the centralised and the distributed approaches.

3 Case Study: Assessment for Breast Cancer

We present as our case study the medical guideline for assessing the presence of breast cancer, because, as we will describe in more detail in the next section, a computer-based, centralised workflow has already been developed, making the comparison easier. This guideline is part of a larger more complex workflow, that includes periodical screening, surgical intervention and follow-up.

Breast cancer is the most commonly diagnosed cancer in women, accounting for about 30% of all such cancers. One in nine women will develop breast cancer at some point in their lives. In the UK, women with symptoms that raise suspicion of breast cancer are referred by their GP to designated breast clinics. To increase the accuracy of diagnosis, a combination of clinical examination, imaging and biopsy - known together as *triple assessment* - is recommended.

The first element of triple assessment consists of gathering the patient details and clinical examinations, and it is completed by a breast surgeon. If the clinical examination reveals an abnormality then the patient is referred to a radiologist for imaging (either ultrasound, mammography or both). If either the examination or imaging findings warrant it, then a biopsy is performed, either by a radiologist or a surgeon, and the tissue is sent to a pathologist for examination. The collective results from all three tests influence the final management of the patient. Depending on the resources available, different imaging and pathology laboratories might be selected every time the guideline is executed, possibly from different institutions.

A small number of 'worried well' patients may not qualify for either imaging or biopsy and could be discharged straight away. As the entire clinical process is distributed among three different disciplines and involves a number of different clinicians, a very close co-ordination and good communication between those involved is essential for the smooth running of the clinic.

4 Centralised and Distributed Models

The triple assessment model presented in [26] is designed according to a centralised principle, and the abstract workflow is shown in Figure 1. The centralised model

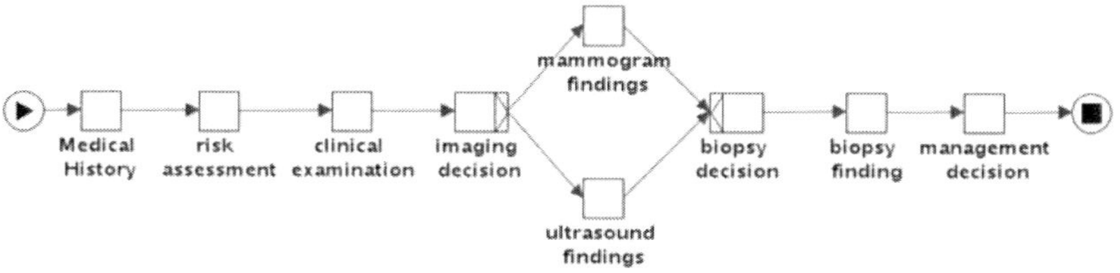

Fig. 1. Centralised representation of the triple assessment

has been implemented[3] in PRO*forma* [31], a process modelling language developed within Cancer Research UK. Together with the possibility of representing plans, sub-plans and actions, its strength lays in its decision support system, based on argumentation.

However, in PRO*forma* it is not possible to explicitly represent different roles in a guideline: roles are enforced by requiring different permissions to access the activities. Activities are queued in the todo list of a user, who is presented with this list after logging in. When the user finishes the activity, it is marked as completed and the workflow proceeds. While PRO*forma* provides a strong support for representing and reasoning about medical knowledge, it is currently inadequate for representing and executing coordinated activities between distributed actors.

The distributed nature of the procedure cannot be reconstructed from its representation as a centralised workflow. Moreover, medical knowledge specific to different participants, that is, the arguments and rules necessary for decisions in various phases, is centralised in a single procedure, making it impossible to reuse the same knowledge in different guidelines. If the model is implemented in another workflow language such as BPEL, the knowledge could be split amongst a group of services, possibly each based on PRO*forma*, but the process itself would still be represented from a single perspective.

A more realistic representation of the flow of the procedure is provided by the UML Activity diagram of Figure 2, in which the participants and their interactions are made explicit. Figure 3 is a corresponding UML Sequence diagram. There are five main actors: the breast surgery service (BSS), in charge of the first three activities in the workflow in Figure 1, the breast imaging service (BIS), responsible for the imaging decision and for the two alternative possible examinations, the breast pathology service (BPS), in charge of the biopsy, the multi-disciplinary team (MDT), responsible for the final decision together with the surgery service, and the patient.

The aim of this work is to allow the distribution of knowledge and information to the actors in charge, the reuse of knowledge in different guidelines, and the possibility of easily adapting guidelines to the realities of actual institutions and hospitals. We obtain this by separating the two different aspects of guidelines into two abstraction layers. The higher level consists in the choreography that specifies the expected

[3] A demo is available at: `http://tinyurl.com/tripleassessment`

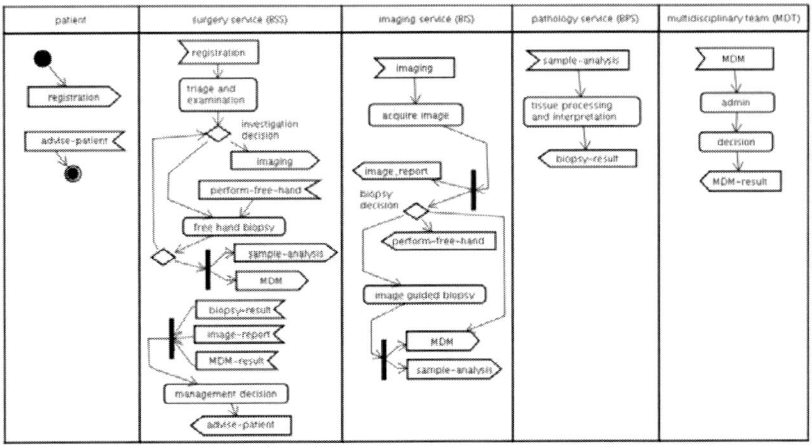

Fig. 2. Activity diagram for the triple assessment

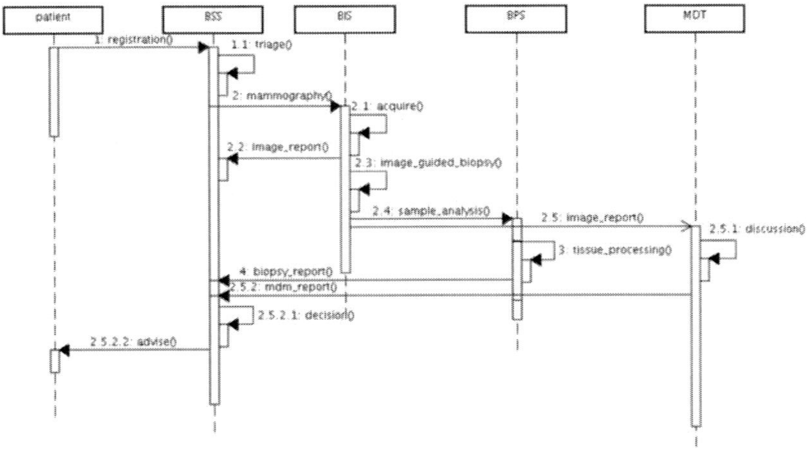

Fig. 3. Fragment of the sequence diagram of a run of the triple assessment

behaviour interface of the participants. The choreography is shared, and the participants agree to follow it. The lower level consists in the specific knowledge and services, local to participants, that are mapped to the choreography. The choreography provides a specific context and the semantics for the interaction, giving the boundaries of the task of integrating the different participants.

5 The OpenKnowledge Approach

5.1 Sharing Choreographies

A choreography-based architecture can help developers to think about distributed applications from a different perspective, one which scales better with an increasing number of interacting actors. A distributed application becomes a set of interactions between actors that assume different roles, their internal behaviour is kept separated from their external behaviour.

In most distributed approaches, the workflow engineer selects the participants: the list of participants is a basic construct both in choreography languages such as WS-CDL [23], BPEL4Chor [11] and in orchestration languages such as BPEL [2]. Some workflow architectures, such as Taverna [22], let the developer specify a list of alternative services to call if the first fails, but the binding is still at design time. Service descriptions are stored in shared repositories and the designer looks up the specific service for a task.

This approach makes portability more difficult. As we have seen, guidelines are usually written by a committee of experts with a view to being generally applicable: when the plan has to be implemented by adopting institutions, it may require heavy customisation to adapt it to their requirements (for example, the list of services to invoke is likely to be different, and therefore part of the specification has to be changed).

In our approach, the choreographies are published in a shared repository, similarly to the publication of a guideline by a committee. Participants search the appropriate choreographies when they need to perform an activity that requires the coordinated activity of other actors. The choreographies are matched against the participants' capabilities: the participants select the choreography that best fit them and advertise their intention to perform a role within a choreography. If all the roles are filled, the interaction can start. In our triple assessment example, this means that roles such as the breast imaging service or the breast pathology service are bound at run time, when the procedure needs to be performed, based on their availability.

We believe that this allows increased reuse both of choreographies and of participants' components, and allows the deployment of distributed applications with different degrees of freedom, maintaining the same architecture. Without altering the architecture presented in this Chapter, it is possible to implement a closed system where for a task there is only one possible choreography and a fixed set of other participants that are bound to it, and an open system where for a task a participant has the freedom of choosing different choreographies, and has a choice between different participants who are free to accept.

In the choreography model, issues of heterogeneity and brokering need to be addressed. Participants are likely to be different and they need to understand one another. The same services may be available from many peers, and the search and discovery process can be complex, especially if it needs to be performed at real time. The OpenKnowledge framework addresses these issues.

5.2 The OpenKnowledge Framework

The OpenKnowledge kernel [30] provides the middleware that assorted services can use to interact using a choreography-based architecture able to deal both with the semantic heterogeneity of the actors and with their discovery. It has been designed with the goals of being lightweight and compact, allowing a short development cycle for distributed applications.

$$
\begin{aligned}
Model &:= \{Clause, \ldots\} \\
Clause &:= Role :: Def \\
Role &:= a(Type, Id) \\
Def &:= Role \mid Message \mid Def\ then\ Def \mid \\
&\quad\ Def\ or\ Def \\
Message &:= M \Rightarrow Role \mid M \Rightarrow Role \leftarrow C \mid \\
&\quad\ M \Leftarrow Role \mid C \leftarrow M \Leftarrow Role \\
C &:= Constant \mid P(Term, \ldots) \mid \neg C \mid C \wedge C \mid \\
&\quad\ C \vee C \\
Type &:= Term \\
Id &:= Constant \mid Variable \\
M &:= Term \\
Term &:= Constant \mid Variable \mid P(Term, \ldots) \\
Constant &:= \text{lower case character sequence or number} \\
Variable &:= \text{upper case character sequence or number}
\end{aligned}
$$

Fig. 4. LCC syntax

The framework allows a direct translation of a choreography oriented design into an executable application. The core concept is the shared *interaction models* (IM), performed by different applications and service providers. These actors are the participants, called *peers*, of the interactions, and they play *roles* in them. In an interaction all the roles have equal weight; the behaviour of all the peers and in particular their exchange of messages are specified.

IMs are written in the Lightweight Coordination Calculus (LCC) [28,29], a compact, executable choreography language based on process calculus. Its syntax is shown in Figure 4. The IMs are published by the authors on the *distributed discovery service* (DDS) with a keyword-based description [24].

An IM in LCC is a contract that defines the expected, externally observable, behavioural interfaces of the roles that participants can take in the interaction: an IM is a set of role clauses. Participants in an interaction take their *entry-role* and follow the unfolding of the clause specified using combinations of the sequence operator

```
a(bss,BSS) ::
registration(P) ⇐ a(patient,P) then
null ← triage(TR,P) and examine(TR,ER,P) then
( null ← isImagingDecision(ER) then
  doImaging(P,TI) ⇒ a(bis,BIS)
     ← typeOfImaging(ER,TI) )
or
( ( ( null ← isFreeHandBiopsy(ER)
      then
      null ← doFreeHandBiopsy(P,FHBR) )
    or
    null ← true )
  then
  ( null ← isBiopsy(ER) then
    doSampleAnalysis(P) ⇒ a(bps,BPS) then
    doMDM(P,TR,ER,FHBR) ⇒ a(mdt,MDT) ) )
then
a(bss_wait_resports([],Reports),BSS)
then
null ← mngmt_decision(P,TR,ER,FHBR,Reports,Dec)
then
advise(Dec) ⇒ a(patient,P)

a(bss_wait_reports(RPT,NewRPT),BSS) ::
null ← all_arrived(RPT) and NewRPT = RPT
or ( biopsy_report(P,BR) ⇐ a(bps,BPS) then
     a(bss_wait_reports([BR|RPT],NewRPT) )
or ( mdm_report(P,MR) ⇐ a(mdt,MDT) then
     a(bss_wait_reports([MR|RPT],NewRPT) )
or ( image_report(P,IR) ⇐ a(bis,BIS) then
     a(bss_wait_reports([IR|RPT],NewRPT) )
```

Fig. 5. LCC clauses for the `breast surgery service(BSS)` role

(‘*then*’) or choice operator (‘*or*’) to connect messages and changes of role. Messages are either outgoing to (‘⇒’) or incoming from (‘⇐’) another participant in a given role. A participant can take, during an interaction, more roles and can recursively take the same role (for example when processing a list). Message input/output or change of role is controlled by constraints. In its definition, LCC makes no commitment to the method used to solve constraints - so different participants might operate different constraint solvers.

Figures 5 and 6 show the LCC clause for the breast surgery service (`BSS`) and the breast imaging service (`BIS`) roles in the triple assessment procedure described in the activity diagram of Figure 2. In the surgery service clause, the participant who takes the `bss` role starts waiting for the registration message from a patient. When the request message arrives, it executes the triage and the examination on the patient. Based on the result of the examination, the surgery service either asks the imaging service to acquire an image, or performs a free hand biopsy, asks the pathologist

$$
\begin{array}{l}
\texttt{a(bis,BIS)} :: \\
\texttt{doImaging(P,TI)} \Leftarrow \texttt{a(bss,BSS) then} \\
\texttt{null} \leftarrow \texttt{acquire\_image(P,TI,IMR) then} \\
\texttt{image\_report(P,IMR)} \Rightarrow \texttt{a(bss\_wait\_reports,BSS)} \\
\texttt{then} \\
\left(\begin{array}{l}
\texttt{null} \leftarrow \texttt{isBiopsyDecision(IMR) then} \\
\texttt{null} \leftarrow \texttt{doBiopsy(P,IMR,S) then} \\
\texttt{doSampleAnalysis(P)} \Rightarrow \texttt{a(bps,BPS) then} \\
\texttt{doMDM(P,TR,ER,FHBR)} \Rightarrow \texttt{a(mdt,MDT)}
\end{array}\right) \\
\texttt{or} \\
\texttt{null} \leftarrow \texttt{true}
\end{array}
$$

Fig. 6. LCC clause for the `breast imaging service (BIS)` role

to analyse the sample, and sends a request for a multi-disciplinary meeting. Then the process changes role, and waits for the reports from the contacted specialists. When all the reports have arrived, the process returns to the main role and makes the decision about the patient.

In the imaging service clause, the actor taking the role starts by waiting for a request `doImaging(P,TI)` from the surgery service. Then it acquires and analyses an image using the method specified in `TI` (either an ultrasound scan, or a mammography), and sends the report to the surgery service. If required it performs a biopsy, asks a pathologist to analyse the sample and sends a report to the multi-disciplinary team for discussion.

Most of the constraints, such as `triage(P,TR)` or `doFreeHandBiopsy (P,FHBR)`, correspond to external activities, that a doctor or a radiologist perform. They may be completed by filling in computerised forms or by receiving data from an external device such as an ultrasound scan machine. Some constraints, such as `acquire(P,TI,IMR)` may launch further interactions (in this case, a different one depending on the method required, and involving a radiologist).

LCC prescribes only the ordering of the exchanged messages and their pre and post-conditions in the form of constraints peers need to solve. However, in OpenKnowledge it is possible to annotate every element in the IM in order to enrich the description of the interaction. Annotations are mainly used to define the ontological type of the variables in messages and constraints, but time-out for messages and constraints could be expressed using the same mechanism. Figure 7 describes the syntax

$$
\begin{aligned}
annotation &:= @annotation(about, innerAnnot) \\
about &:= @role(Role)|@message(M)| \\
&\quad\ @constraint(Term)| \\
&\quad\ @variable(Variable) \\
innerAnnot &:= annotation|tree \\
tree &:= Constant|tree|Constant, tree
\end{aligned}
$$

Fig. 7. Annotations syntax

Constraint annotations
```
@annotation(@role(bss),
  @annotation(@variable(TR),
   risk_level)
)
@annotation(@role(bss),
  @annotation(@variable(P),
   patient(name,surname,date_of_birth,
    address(street,post_code)) )
)
```

Java method annotation
```
@MethodSemantic(language=''tag'',
params={
  ''patient(family_name,birthday,street,post_code)'',
  ''risk(assessed_level,confidence)''
})
public boolean doTriage(Argument P,
          Argument TR)
{...}
```

Fig. 8. Annotations for the constraint *triage(P,TR)* and for a corresponding method

used in annotations. An example of annotation for the variables in role `bss` is shown in Figure 8. This specific example shows how variables can be structured terms: the variable *P* is, in the choreography, the structure `patient(name,surname, date_of_birth, address(street,post_code)))`. The structure is a short-hand for an XML-like schema, where the functions and the parameters are nested tags in a tree. Annotations are always relative to a specific role-clause in the interaction: the scope of a variable is always limited to a clause.

Annotations are conceptually separated from the IM itself. It is possible to attach different annotations to the same IM to adapt it to different requirements and contexts: for example, the same abstract IM could be used in a different community, that specifies patients by their insurance numbers, and therefore annotates variable *P* differently.

A peer that wants to perform some task, such as providing an imaging service for breast cancer screening, searches for published IMs for the task by sending a keyword-based query to the DDS. The DDS collects the published IMs matching the description (the keywords are extended adding synonyms to improve recall) and sends the list back to the peer, that needs to choose the one to subscribe.

In open systems, IMs and peers may be designed by different entities, and therefore the constraints and the peers' knowledge bases are unlikely to correspond perfectly. The heterogeneity problem is dealt with in three phases. We have already seen the first phase: the DDS matches the interaction descriptions using a simple query expansion mechanism. Then the peers compare the constraints in the received IMs with their own capabilities [20], and finally the peers need to map the terms appearing in constraints and introduced by other peers [9]. The scope of the matching problem is limited to the specific IM in the second phase, and to the specific interaction run in the third phase.

The peer capabilities are provided by plug-in components, called OKCs (Open-Knowledge Components) that can be published by the developers on the DDS and downloaded by other peers. An OKC exposes a set of Java methods that are compared to the constraints in the IMs. The arguments of methods can be annotated similarly to variables in the IM. Arguments, like variables in constraints, can be structured terms. Figure 8 shows an annotated method with structured arguments. As annotations are short-hands for XML-like trees, values in an argument are accessed by their path, similarly to a very simplified XPath: for example, to obtain the street of a patient, the method `doTriage` will call the method `getValue(''/street'')` of the argument P.

The peer matches the annotated signatures of the constraints and of the methods, transforming them into trees and verifying their distance [15,20]. The comparison process creates *adaptors*, that bridge the constraints to the methods, as shown in Figure 9. An adaptor has a confidence level, reflecting the distance between the constraints and the matching method, that gives a measure of how well the peer can execute an interaction, and it used to select the most fitting IM. Once the peer has selected an IM, it subscribes to its role in the discovery service. Figure 10 shows a snapshot of network status when roles in an interaction are subscribed by at least one peer.

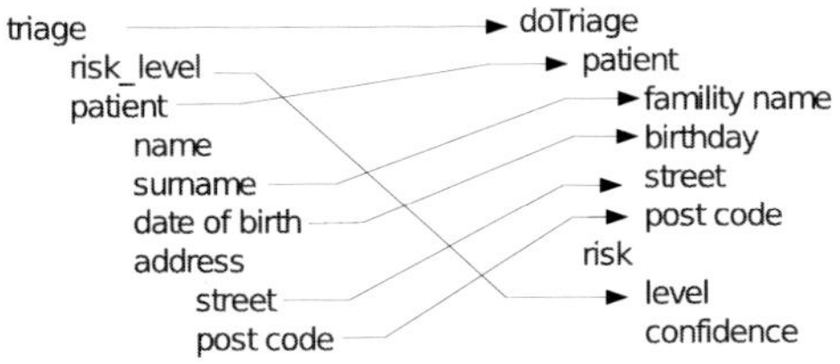

Fig. 9. Adaptor for constraint *deliver(M,P)*

When all the roles are filled, the discovery service chooses randomly a peer in the network as coordinator for the interaction, and hands over the IM together with the list of involved peers in order to execute it.

The coordinator first asks each peer to select the peers they want to interact with, forming a mutually compatible group of peers out of the replies. The selection process is subjective to the peers. All the participants receive the list of peers subscribed to all the roles, and they can check the subscriptions, selecting the preferred ones. A peer can also select none of the participants, excluding itself from a particular run of the interaction, for instance due to overload. The framework provides only an interface for the selection method, as its implementation is delegated to the application developer. However, different strategies have been tested, as we will see in the evaluation section.

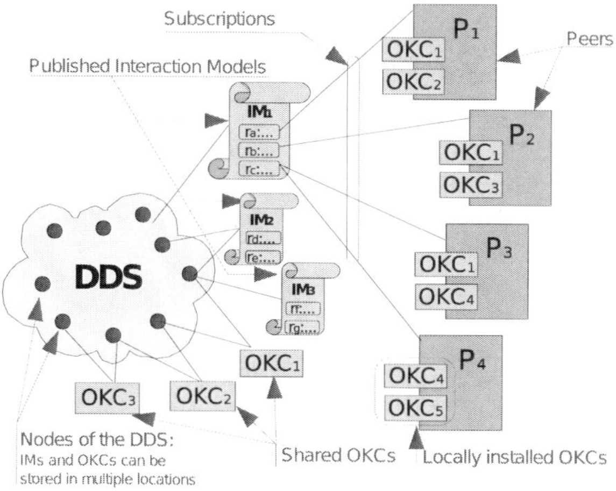

Fig. 10. OpenKnowledge architecture

While different implementations are possible, in the current version of the OpenKnowledge kernel the coordinator executes the interaction, instantiating a local proxy for each peer. The remote peers are contacted only to solve constraints in the role they have subscribed.

6 Related Work

This Section discusses all related work from the literature, spanning pure choreography languages, enhancements to widely used modelling techniques, i.e. BPMN, decentralised orchestration, data flow optimisation architectures and Grid toolkits.

6.1 Choreography Languages

The majority of workflow research has focused on designing languages for and implementing service orchestrations, from the view of a single participant. Examples can be seen in the Business Process Modelling community through BPEL [32] and life sciences community through Taverna [25]. However, there are relatively few languages targeted specifically at service choreography, the most widely known are:

• WS-CDL: The Web Services Choreography Description Language (WS-CDL) is the proposed standard for service choreography, currently at the W3C Candidate Recommendation stage. However, WS-CDL has met criticism [7,13] through the Web services community. It is not within the scope of this Chapter to provide a detailed analysis of the constructs of WS-CDL, this research has already been presented [17]. However, it is useful to point out the key criticisms with the language: WS-CDL choreographies are tightly bound to specific WSDL interfaces, WS-CDL has no multi-party support, no agreed formal foundation, no explicit graphical support and few or incomplete implementations.

• Let's Dance [36]: is a language that supports service interaction modelling both from a global and local viewpoint. In a global (or choreography) model, interactions are described from the viewpoint of an ideal observer who oversees all interactions between a set of services. Local models, on the other hand focus on the perspective of a particular service, capturing only those interactions that directly involve it. Using Let's Dance, a choreography consists of a set of interrelated service interactions which correspond to message exchanges. Communication is performed by an actor playing a role. Interaction is specified using one of three Let's Dance constructs: *precedes* – the source interaction can only occur after the target interaction has occurred; *inhibits* – denotes that after the source interaction has occurred, the target interaction can no longer occur, and finally *weak precedes* – denotes that the target interaction can only occur after the source interaction has reached a final status, e.g. completed or skipped. A complete overview of the Let's Dance language is presented in [36], including solutions to the Service Interaction Patterns [8].

• BPEL4Chor [12]: is a proposal for adding an additional layer to BPEL to shift its emphasis from an orchestration language to a complete choreography language. BPEL4Chor is a simple, collection of three artifact types: *participant behaviour descriptions* define the control flow dependencies between activities, in particular between communication activities, at a given participant. A *participant topology* describes the structural aspects of a choreography by specifying participant types, participant references and message links; this serves as the glue between the participant behaviour descriptions. Finally *participant groundings* define the technical configuration details, the choreography becomes Web service specific, concrete links to WSDL definitions and XSD types are established. BPEL4Chor is an effective proposal and importantly conforms to standards [4] by enhancing the industrially supported BPEL specification. BPEL4Chor encourages reuse by only providing a specific Web service mapping in the participant grounding. Furthermore, unknown numbers of participants can be modelled, not possible with WS-CDL.

6.2 Modelling Support

There are several proposals for extending the Business Process Modelling Notation [1]; the de-facto standard for business process modelling. Although the BPMN allows an engineer to define choreographies through a swim lane concept and a distinction between control flow and message flow, it only provides direct support for a limited set of the Service Interaction Patterns and not some of the more advanced choreography scenarios. [10] introduces a set of extensions for BPMN which facilitate an interaction modelling approach as opposed to modelling interconnected interface behaviour models. Authors claim that choreography designers can understand models more effectively, introduce less errors and build models more efficiently. Evaluation concludes that the majority of the Service Interaction Patterns can be expressed with the additional extensions. [14] discusses the deficiencies of the BPMN for choreography modelling and proposes a number of direct extensions for the BPMN which overcome these limitations.

6.3 Techniques in Data Flow Optimisation

There are a limited number of research papers which have identified the problems associated with centralised service orchestration. For completeness, this Section presents an overview of a number of architectures.

• Service Invocation Triggers [37] are also a response to the problem of centralised orchestration engines when dealing with large-scale data sets. Triggers collect the required input data before they invoke a service, forwarding the results directly to where the data is required. For this decentralised execution to take place, a workflow must be deconstructed into sequential fragments which contain neither loops nor conditionals and the data dependancies must be encoded within the triggers themselves. Before execution can begin the input workflow must be deconstructed into sequential fragments, which cannot contain loops and must be installed at a trigger.

• The *Circulate* Architecture [6] maintains the robustness and simplicity of centralised orchestration, but facilitates choreography by allowing services to exchange data directly with one another. Performance analysis [5] concludes that a substantial reduction in communication overhead results in a 2–4 fold performance benefit across all workflow patterns. An end-to-end pattern through the Montage workflow (a benchmark for the HPC community) results in an 8 fold performance benefit and demonstrates how the advantage of using the architecture increases as the complexity of a workflow grows.

• Decentralised Web Service Orchestrations Using WS-BPEL. In [38] the scalability argument made in this paper is also identified. The authors propose a methodology for transforming the orchestration logic in BPEL into a set of individual activities that coordinate themselves by passing tokens over shared, distributed tuple spaces. The model suitable for execution is called Executable Workow Networks (EWFN), a Petri nets dialect.

• Triana [39] is an open-source problem solving environment. It is designed to define, process, analyse, manage, execute and monitor workflows. Triana can distribute sections of a workflow to remote machines through a connected peer-to-peer network. *OGSA-DAI [40]* middleware supports the exposure of data resources on to Grids and facilitates data streaming between local OGSA-DAI instances. *Grid Services Flow Language (GSFL) [41]* addresses some of the issues discussed in this paper in the context of Grid services, in particular services adopt a peer-to-peer data flow model.

7 Conclusion and Future Work

In this Chapter we have argued that a distributed, choreography-based paradigm has a number of practical benefits when applied to design and implementation of complex systems, such as distributed clinical workflows. The choreography paradigm provides a clean approach to issues of portability of workflow specification (allowing a high-level guideline to be implemented at different sites which are likely to have different local procedures for carrying out tasks within the guideline), re-use of process specifications (allowing site-specific implementation detail to be re-used within different high-level process specifications), and abstraction away from the specific entities providing services, which might change both between sites and between runs of the process.

OpenKnowledge provides an operational framework for quickly setting up such systems. In OpenKnowledge, systems are composed around interaction models that coordinate the peers' behaviours by specifying the roles they can take, the exchange of messages between the roles and the constraints of the messages. Peers participate in the interaction taking one (or more) roles: in order to participate they need to compare the constraint in the roles with their available services and subscribe to the interaction on a distributed discovery service, that initiates interactions when their roles are filled.

In the current version of OpenKnowledge, constraints in the choreography are semantically matched with the capabilities of the peers. However, while feasible using the annotations, there is still no support for specifying requirements on how the constraints should be solved, or on what requirements the participants should have (for example, the peer taking the doctor role should be certified by the competent institution). Improving the specifications can help the peers both in selecting the proper interactions for their goals and in matching their capabilities with those required by the choreography.

References

1. Business Process Modeling Notation (BPMN) Specification. Technical report, Object Management Group, OMG (2006), `http://www.omg.org/spec/BPMN/1.1/PDF`
2. Web services business process execution language version 2.0 (April 2007)
3. Anadiotis, G., Kotoulas, S., Lausen, H., Siebes, R.: Massively scalable web service discovery. In: Proceedings of the 23rd Intl. Conference on Advanced Information Networking and Applications, AINA 2009 (2009)
4. Barker, A., van Hemert, J.: Scientific Workflow: A Survey and Research Directions. In: Wyrzykowski, R., et al. (eds.) PPAM 2007. LNCS, vol. 4967, pp. 746–753. Springer, Heidelberg (2008)
5. Barker, A., Weissman, J.B., van Hemert, J.: Eliminating the Middle Man: Peer-to-Peer Dataflow. In: HPDC 2008: Proceedings of the 17th International Symposium on High Performance Distributed Computing, pp. 55–64. ACM, New York (June 2008)
6. Barker, A., Weissman, J.B., van Hemert, J.: Orchestrating Data-Centric Workflows. In: The 8th IEEE International Symposium on Cluster Computing and the Grid (CCGrid), pp. 210–217. IEEE Computer Society, Los Alamitos (May 2008)
7. Barros, A., Dumas, M., Oaks, P.: A Critical Overview of the Web Services Choreography Description Language (WS-CDL). BPTrends Newsletter 3 (March 2005)
8. Barros, A., Dumas, M., ter Hofstede, A.: Service Interaction Patterns. In: van der Aalst, W.M.P., Benatallah, B., Casati, F., Curbera, F. (eds.) BPM 2005. LNCS, vol. 3649, pp. 302–318. Springer, Heidelberg (2005)

9. Besana, P., Robertson, D.: How service choreography statistics reduce the ontology mapping problem. In: Aberer, K., Choi, K.-S., Noy, N., Allemang, D., Lee, K.-I., Nixon, L.J.B., Golbeck, J., Mika, P., Maynard, D., Mizoguchi, R., Schreiber, G., Cudré-Mauroux, P. (eds.) ASWC 2007 and ISWC 2007. LNCS, vol. 4825, pp. 44–57. Springer, Heidelberg (2007)
10. Decker, G., Barros, A.: Interaction Modeling Using BPMN. In: CBP 2007. LNCS, vol. 4928, pp. 206–217. Springer, Heidelberg (2007)
11. Decker, G., Kopp, O., Leymann, F., Weske, M.: BPEL4Chor: extending BPEL for modeling choreographies. In: Society, I.C. (ed.) Proceedings of the IEEE 2007 International Conference on Web Services (ICWS 2007), Salt Lake City, Utah, USA, pp. 296–303. IEEE Computer Society, Los Alamitos (July 2007)
12. Decker, G., Kopp, O., Leymann, F., Weske, M.: BPEL4Chor: Extending BPEL for Modeling Choreographies. In: Proceedings of the IEEE 2007 International Conference on Web Services (ICWS 2007), pp. 296–303 (2007)
13. Decker, G., Overdick, H., Zaha, J.M.: On the Suitability of WS-CDL for Choreography Modeling. In: Proceedings of Methoden, Konzepte und Technologien für die Entwicklung von dienstebasierten Informationssystemen (EMISA), LNI P-95, Hamburg, Germany, pp. 21–34 (October 2006)
14. Decker, G., Puhlmann, F.: Extending BPMN for Modeling Complex Choreographies. In: Meersman, R., Tari, Z. (eds.) OTM 2007, Part I. LNCS, vol. 4803, pp. 24–40. Springer, Heidelberg (2007)
15. F., G., M., Y., F., M.: Structure preserving semantic matching. In: Proceedings of the ISWC+ASWC International workshop on Ontology Matching (OM), Busan, KR (2007)
16. Grimshaw, J.M., Russel, I.T.: Effect of clinical guidelines on medical practice: a systematic review of rigorous evaluations. Lancet 342, 1317–1322 (1993)
17. Fredlund, L.: Implementing WS-CDL. In: Proceedings of the second Spanish workshop on Web Technologies (JSWEB 2006), Universidade de Santiago de Compostela (November 2006)
18. Fox, J., Patkar, V., Thompson, R.: Decision support for health care: the proforma evidence base. Journal of Informatics in Primary Care 14(1), 49–54 (2006)
19. Garg, A., Adhikari, N., McDonald, H., Rosas-Arellano, P., Devereaux, P., Beyene, J., Sam, J., Haynes, R.: Effects of computerised clinical decision support systems on practictioner performance and patient outcome: a systematic review. JAMA 293, 1223–1238 (2005)
20. Giunchiglia, F., McNeill, F., Yatskevich, M., Pane, J., Besana, P., Shvaiko, P.: Approximate structure preserving semantic matching. In: On the Move to Meaningful Internet Systems: OTM 2008, pp. 1217–1234 (2008)
21. Grimshaw, J., Russel, I.: Effect of clinical guidelines on medical practice: A systematic review of rigorous evaluations. Lancet 342, 1317–1322 (1993)
22. Hull, D., Wolstencroft, K., Stevens, R., Goble, C., Pocock, M.R., Li, P., Oinn, T.: Taverna: a tool for building and running workflows of services. Nucleic Acids Res. 34(Web Server issue), W729–W732 (2006)
23. Kavantzas, N., Burdett, D., Ritzinge, G., Fletcher, T., Lafon, Y., Barreto, C.: Web services choreography description language version 1.0 (November 2005), `http://www.w3.org/TR/2005/CR-ws-cdl-10-20051109/`
24. Kotoulas, S., Siebes, R.: Deliverable 2.2: Adaptive routing in structured peer-to-peer overlays. Technical report, OpenKnowledge
25. Oinn, T., Addis, M., Ferris, J., Marvin, D., Senger, M., Greenwood, M., Carver, T., Glover, K., Pocock, M.R., Wipat, A., Li, P.: Taverna: a tool for the composition and enactment of bioinformatics workflows. Bioinformatics 20, 3045–3054 (2004)

26. Patkar, V., Hurt, C., Steele, R., Purushotham, A., Williams, M., Thomson, R., Fox, J.: Evidence-based guidelines and decision support services: a discussion and evaluation in triple assessment of suspected breast cancer. British Journal of Cancer 95, 1490–1496 (2006)
27. Perreau de Pinninck, A., Sierra, C., Walton, C., De la Cruz, D., Robertson, D., Gerloff, D., Jaen, E., Li, Q., Sharman, J., Abian, J., Schorlemmer, M., Besana, P., Leung, S., Quan, X.: D6.4: Summative report on bioinformatics case studies. Technical report, University of Edinburgh (2008)
28. Robertson, D.: Multi-agent coordination as distributed logic programming. In: International Conference on Logic Programming, Sant-Malo, France (2004)
29. Robertson, D., Walton, C., Barker, A., Besana, P., Chen-Burger, Y., Hassan, F., Lambert, D., Li, G., McGinnis, J., Osman, N., Bundy, A., McNeill, F., van Harmelen, F., Sierra, C., Giunchiglia, F.: Models of interaction as a grounding for peer to peer knowledge sharing. In: Advances in Web Semantics I: Ontologies, Web Services and Applied Semantic Web, vol. 4891, pp. 81–129 (2009)
30. Siebes, R., Dupplaw, D., Kotoulas, S., de Pinninck, A.P., van Harmelen, F., Robertson, D.: The openknowledge system: an interaction-centered approach to knowledge sharing. In: Proceedings of the 15th Intl. Conference on Cooperative Information Systems, CoopIS (2007)
31. Sutton, R., Fox, J.: The syntax and semantics of the proforma guideline modeling language. Journal of the American Medical Informatics Association 10(5), 433–443 (2003)
32. The OASIS Committee: Web Services Business Process Execution Language (WS-BPEL) Version 2.0 (2007)
33. Trecarichi, G., Rizzi, V., Vaccari, L., Marchese, M., Besana, P.: Openknowledge at work: exploring centralized and decentralized information gathering in emergency contexts. In: ISCRAM 2009 (2009)
34. Vaccari, L., Shvaiko, P., Marchese, M.: An emergent semantics approach to semantic integration of geo-services and geo-metadata in spatial data infrastructures. International Journal of Spatial Data Infrastructured Research 4, 24–51 (2009)
35. var der Aalst, W., Aldred, L., Dumas, M., ter Hofstede, A.H.M.: Design and implementation of the yawl system. In: Persson, A., Stirna, J. (eds.) CAiSE 2004. LNCS, vol. 3084, pp. 142–159. Springer, Heidelberg (2004)
36. Zaha, J.M., Barros, A., Dumas, M., ter Hofstede, A.: Let's Dance: A Language for Service Behavior Modelling. In: Meersman, R., Tari, Z. (eds.) OTM 2006. LNCS, vol. 4275, pp. 145–162. Springer, Heidelberg (2006)
37. Binder, W., Constantinescu, I., Faltings, B.: Decentralized Ochestration of Composite Web Services. In: Proccedings of the International Conference on Web Services, ICWS 2006, pp. 869–876. IEEE Computer Society, Los Alamitos (2006)
38. Martin, D., Wutke, D., Leymann, F.: A Novel Approach to Decentralized Workflow Enactment. In: EDOC 2008. 12th International IEEE Conference on Enterprise Distributed Object Computing, pp. 127–136 (2008)
39. Taylor, I., Shields, M., Wang, I., Philp, R.: Distributed P2P Computing within Triana: A Galaxy Visualization Test Case. In: 17th International Parallel and Distributed Processing Symposium (IPDPS 2003), pp. 16–27. IEEE Computer Society, Los Alamitos (2003)
40. Karasavvas, K., Antonioletti, M., Atkinson, M., Hong, N.C., Sugden, T., Hume, A., Jackson, M., Krause, A., Palansuriya, C.: Introduction to OGSA-DAI Services. In: Herrero, P., S. Pérez, M., Robles, V. (eds.) SAG 2004. LNCS, vol. 3458, pp. 1–12. Springer, Heidelberg (2005)
41. Krishnan, S., Wagstrom, P., Laszewski, G.v.: GSFL: A Workflow Framework for Grid Services. Technical report, Argonne National Argonne National Laboratory (2002)

Chapter 4
Data Mining Based on Intelligent Systems for Decision Support Systems in Healthcare

Loris Nanni[1], Sheryl Brahnam[2], Alessandra Lumini[1], and Tonya Barrier[2]

[1] DEIS, IEIIT—CNR, Università di Bologna,
Viale Risorgimento 2, 40136 Bologna, Italy
loris.nanni@unibo.it, alessandra.lumini@unibo.it
[2] Computer Information Systems, Missouri State University,
901 S. National, Springfield, MO 65804, USA
sbrahnam@missouristate.edu
tonyabarrier@missouristate.edu

Abstract. In this paper we make an extensive study of Artificial Intelligence (AI) techniques that can be used in decision support systems in healthcare. In particular, we propose variants of ensemble methods (i.e., Rotation Forest and Input Decimated Ensembles) that are based on perturbing features, and we make a wide comparison among the ensemble approaches. We illustrate the power of these techniques by applying our approaches to different healthcare problems. Included in this chapter is extensive background material on the single classifier systems, ensemble methods, and feature transforms used in the experimental section.

Keywords: rotation forest, input decimated ensembles, multiclassifier systems, decision trees, medical decision support systems.

1 Introduction

Across the globe, healthcare is suffering from financial pressures. When making healthcare decisions, administrators and physicians must analyze both clinical and financial information. Many organizations are asking how they can address the problem of maintaining quality healthcare while simultaneously lowering costs to remain competitive. To address this problem, healthcare organizations are starting to make extensive use of state-of-the-art data mining technologies.

Data mining uses advanced statistical methods, database technology, artificial intelligence, pattern recognition, machine learning, and data visualization to discover hidden patterns in data. Two potential uses of data mining in medicine that could reduce costs significantly include predicting patient reactions to drugs and identifying patients who might best benefit from adjuvant chemotherapy (by comparing, for example, patients who continue to be disease free after five years with patients who develop metastases within five years). By properly managing patients today, tomorrow's problems and costs can be reduced. It may soon be

S. Brahnam & L.C. Jain (Eds.): Adv. Comput. Intell. Paradigms in Healthcare 5, SCI 326, pp. 45–65.
springerlink.com

possible, given the rise of telemedicine, for data mining methods to be stored on centralized servers accessible to physicians around the world. By submitting relevant information about patients and outcomes, servers would be able to offer expert recommendations that could continuously be refined. In these and other ways, data mining has the potential of helping healthcare organizations achieve their goal of maximizing quality care while minimizing costs.

With scientists continuously producing more information than can be processed, a phenomenon frequently referred to as data avalanche, the potential offered by data mining will only continue to grow. What needs to be developed today to begin realizing this potential are new classification methods that are highly flexible and that offer reasonable accuracy in prediction. In other words, we need general purpose classification methods that are capable of handling a wide variety of medical problems, that compare well with human expertise, and that compete with less flexible state-of-the-art methods that have been crafted for very specific problems. In addition, these new classification methods need to be able to integrate the multiple sources of data that define medical problems, such as data that is derived from clinical protocols, laboratory measurements, and features extracted from signals and images.

Some recent research that approaches some of these broader goals include the work of [2, 9, 18, 24, 27]. One of the most promising techniques for improving both the flexibility and the accuracy of classification systems is to build systems that combine multiple classifiers [15]. The main idea behind a multiclassifier system is to average the hypotheses of a diverse group of classifiers, for instance, an ensemble of classifiers, in order to produce a better approximation to a true hypothesis [13]. In the last few years, a number of methods have been proposed in the literature for building multiclassifier systems.

In this chapter we provide an extensive review and evaluation of muliticlassifier techniques that can be reasonably used in data mining and in building practical decision support systems in healthcare. In section 2 we describe several methods for constructing ensembles of classifiers. We also describe state-of-the-art stand-alone classifiers (such as support vector machines, neural networks, and Gaussian process classifiers) that perform well on specific problems or, in the case of the Gaussian process classifier, in ensembles. Also included in this section is a description of some of the best feature transforms for extracting relevant information from noise. In section 3, we present our ensemble methods, using Rotation Forest, Input Decimated Ensemble, and rotation boosting that are based on variants of the feature transforms. In section 4, we describe several benchmark databases that provide a wide range of different kinds of medical data. In section 5, we apply our ensemble methods to these databases to illustrate the flexibility and accuracy of multiclassifier methods. Specifically, we compare several variants of the ensemble methods by varying the feature transform used to project the patterns. We also vary the method for selecting a set of training patterns for calculating the projections. We compare the results of our multiclassifier systems to the best stand-alone systems. Finally, in section 6, we summarize our results and make suggestions for further research.

2 Multiclassifier Systems

As illustrated in Fig. 1, the basic idea of a simple stand-alone classifier system is to take inputs (from a sensor, for example), preprocess and transform that input to reduce noise and enhance correlation in the data, extract pertinent features, and then adjust the classifier parameters so that the classifier optimally learns from a training set to assign predefined labels to unknown samples in a testing set.

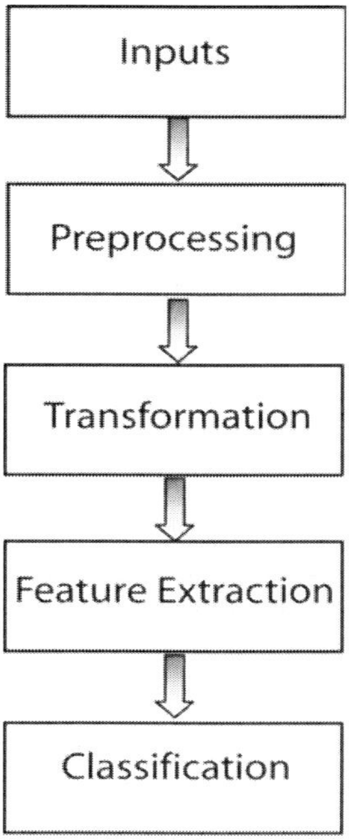

Fig. 1. General outline of a standalone classification system

The basic idea of a multiclassifier system, as illustrated in Fig. 2, is to construct a set of classifiers from the training data that predict class labels from previously unseen records in the testing set by aggregating predictions made by an ensemble of classifiers. There are several methods for aggregating, or combining, the decisions of multiple classifiers. The most common methods are majority voting, sum rule, max rule, min rule, product rule, median rule, and Borda count. The sum rule (averaging) has been shown to outperform most combination rules [13].

Multiclassifier systems are constructed by dividing or perturbing the patterns or the features in the training set, as seen in Fig. 2. It is also possible to focus on the classifiers by combining the results of different classifier types or by perturbing the parameters of a set of classifiers of the same type. Combinations of these methods, or hybrid systems, are also possible. Below we discuss each of these possibilities.

The basic steps involved in constructing multiclassifier systems by perturbing either the patterns or the features in the original training set are the following:

Step 1: Generate K new training sets starting from the original training set;
Step 2: Train a different classifier for each of the K new training sets;
Step 3: Combine the K classifiers using a decision rule.

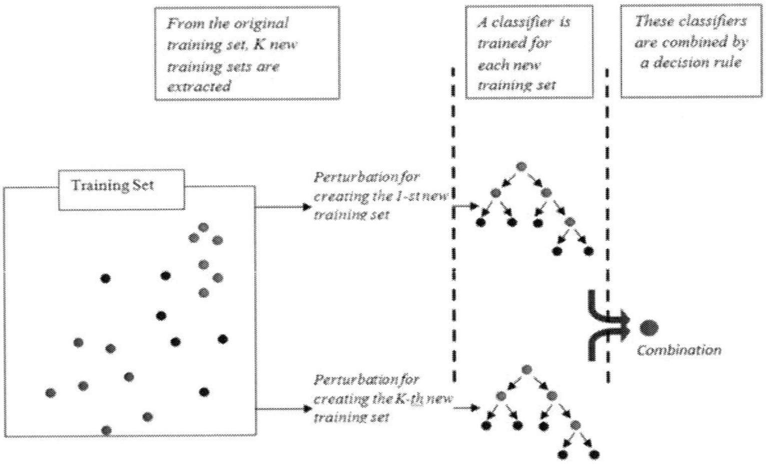

Fig. 2. A multiclassifier system constructed by perturbing either the patterns or the features of the training set

In pattern perturbation, new training sets are constructed by changing the patterns in the original training set. Oftentimes this is done iteratively. Some common methods for constructing new training sets include Bagging [3], where new training sets, $S_1,\ldots, S_K$, are subsets of the original training set; Arcing [2], where misclassified patterns are used to calculate the patterns included in each new training set; Class Switching [20], where K training sets are randomly created by changing the labels of a subset of the training set; Decorate [21], where the training sets are constructed by the addition of patterns that the combined decision of the multiclassifier system misclassifies; Boosting/AdaBoost [7], where each training pattern is given a weight that increases at each iteration for those patterns that are most difficult to classify; and Clusterization [23], where new training sets, $S_1,\ldots, S_K$, are obtained by considering the membership of the training patterns of the clusters found by Fuzzy C-Means.

In feature perturbation,[1] new training sets are created by changing the feature set. Some common methods for perturbing features include Random Subspace [11], where new training sets, $S_1,\ldots, S_K$, are subsets of the feature set; Cluster-based Pattern Discrimination [22], where new training sets, $S_1,\ldots, S_K$, are built by independently partitioning the classes into clusters and then defining different features for each cluster; Input Decimated Ensemble [35], where the new training set S_i is obtained using the principal component analysis (PCA) transform calculated on the training patterns that belong to class *i*. It should be noted that in Input Decimated Ensemble, the size of the ensemble is bounded by the number of classes. This drawback is avoided in [26, 27], where the training patterns are partitioned into clusters, and the PCA transform is then performed on the training patterns within each cluster. Some additional methods of feature perturbation include [31], where four neural networks are trained on different encoding models for identifying Escherichia coli promoter sequences in strings of DNA. In [24], training sets are built using different physicochemical properties of amino acids that are selected using Sequential Forward Floating Selection [30]. Finally, in [8] each classifier is trained using different feature extraction methods.

In classification perturbation different classifiers or classifiers of the same type but with various parameter values are trained on the same training set and the decisions are combined. In [24], for instance, the weights of each classifier are determined by a genetic algorithm. Examples of systems that combine different types of classifiers include [16], where five different classifiers (Logistic Regression, Linear Discriminant Analysis, Quadratic Discriminant Analysis, Naive Bayes, and K-Nearest Neighbors) are combined, using a weighted-vote decision rule to predict which genes respond to stress; and in [25], where three radically different classifiers, a linear Support Vector Machine, a nonlinear radial-basis Support Vector Machine, and a Karhunen-Loeve Subspace, are combined and used to solve a wide variety of classification problems.

Hybrid methods combine different perturbation methods for constructing multiclassifier systems. Some examples include Random Forest [4], which is a bagging ensemble of Decision Trees, where a random selection of features are used to split a given node; Rotation Forest [33], which is an ensemble of Decision Trees where the new training sets, $S_1,\ldots, S_K$, are constructed by applying several PCA projections on subsets of the training patterns. A number of papers have also reported the value of using Independent Component Analysis (ICA) as a feature transform for building a rotation forest ensemble, see, for example, [18, 26, 27]. RotBoost [40] is a method for constructing an ensemble of Decision Trees that combines Rotation Forest and Adaboost. In [40], RotBoost is shown to outperform Bagging, MultiBoost, Rotation Forest, and AdaBoost.

For an excellent tutorial on ensemble methods, we recommend reading Kuncheva's book [14]. For general books on machine learning, pattern recognition and classification, Alpaydin [1], Duda, Hart and Stork [6], and Russell and Norvig [34] provide good overviews.

---

[1] Few general purpose methods of feature perturbation have been proposed, in part because features are specific to problem models. For this reason, we review several papers that propose a system that solves specific problems.

3 System Architecture

Since the aim of this chapter is to compare several variants of ensemble methods that are based mostly on feature perturbation methods (Rotation Forest, Input Decimated Ensemble, and Rotation Boosting), this section provides a more detailed description of these and the other ensemble methods used in our experiments. Each of these perturbation methods was coupled with four different methods of feature transformation, as discussed in section 3.2. The classifier used in our ensembles, is the decision tree. We chose it because of its instability. It is well known that unstable classifiers perform best in ensembles [14]. In section 3.3, we provide a detailed description of decision trees. We also include a brief description of the stand-alone classifiers used in our comparisons, *viz.*, Support Vector Machines, Levenberg-Marquardt Neural Networks (LMNN), and the Gaussian Process Classifier.

3.1 System Ensemble Methods

In this subsection we provide a general discussion, followed by an algorithmic outline, of the ensemble methods used in our experiments.

3.1.1 Bagging

The term bagging is an acronym for Bootstrap AGGregatING, an ensemble method that was first proposed in [3]. The main idea of bagging is to generate random bootstrap training subsets, with replacement, from the original training set. A classifier is then trained on each of these subsets and the results of the classifiers are combined. Bagging is motivated by the fact that the pools of new training sets produce results that are less variant statistically and by the fact that the combined decision made by the system is more tolerant of errors introduced by outliers.

Success using this method is dependent on the selection of the base classifier. To guarantee diversity, the classifier needs to be unstable so that small variations in the training set produce large changes in the classifiers. If the classifiers are not unstable, the ensemble will perform no better than the individual classifiers.

Outline of Bagging

Below is a simple pseudocode description of the bagging algorithm.

In the training process:

For t = 1, 2, …T do:

1. Build a random subset $\mathbf{x}_t$ taking randomly selected samples from the original training set;
2. Train a classifier C_t using the subset $\mathbf{x}_t$;
3. Add the classifier to the ensemble.

In the testing process:

Build the final decision rule by combining the results of the classifiers. Several decision rules can be used to combine the classifiers, e.g., majority voting, the sum rule, and the max rule [13]. In our experiments we use the sum rule.

3.1.2 Random Subspace

Random Subspace [11] (RS) is a method for reducing dimensionality by randomly sampling subsets of features (50% of all the features in our experiments). RS modifies the training data set by generating K (K=50 in our experiments) new training sets. It builds classifiers on these modified training sets. In other words, each classifier is trained on each of the new training sets. The results are combined using the sum rule.

Outline of Random Subspace

As outlined in [11], the random subspace ensemble method is characterized by three steps:

1. Given a *d*-dimensional data set D = $\{(x_j, t_j) \mid 1 \leq j \leq m\}, x_j \in X \subset \mathbb{R}^d$, $t_j \in$ C= $\{1,...,c\}$, *n* new projected *k*-dimensional data sets D_i = $\{(P_i(x_j), t_j) \mid 1 \leq j \leq m\}$ are generated $(1 \leq i \leq n)$, where P_i is a random projection $P_i : \mathbb{R}^d \to \mathbb{R}^k$. P_i is obtained by random selecting, through the uniform probability distribution, a *k*-subset $A = \{\alpha_1, ..., \alpha_k\}$ from $\{1, 2, ..., d\}$ and setting $P_i(x_i, ..., x_d) = (x_{\alpha 1}, ..., x_{\alpha k})$;
2. Each new data set t D_i is given in input to a fixed learning algorithm L which outputs the classifiers h_i for all $i, 1 \leq 1 \leq n$;
3. The final classifier *h* is obtained by aggregating the base classifiers $h_i, ..., h_n$ through a given decision rule.

3.1.3 Rotation Forest

Rotation Forest, proposed in [33], combines the idea of using different feature transforms with the idea of perturbing the training patterns and features. As noted in section 2, it is a method for building ensembles from independently trained decision trees. It has been found to be more accurate as a general method than bagging, AdaBoost, and Random Forest [40].

Outline of Rotation Forest

Let **T** be a training set containing *Q* samples and let **F** be the feature set. Furthermore, let $T_i \in \Re^F$ and let D_i be the *i*-th classifier of the ensemble.

Given a dimension *M*, subsets of *M* features are extracted from **F** (see [33] for details). For each of these subsets a random subset of classes and a bootstrap of samples are extracted. Various feature transforms, such as PCA, ICA, or Neighborhood Preserving Embedding (NPE), are calculated using the selected training patterns. The projections calculated for each subset of *M* features are then combined to build a projection matrix that is used to build a modified training set. The set of classifiers trained on the modified training sets is combined using the sum rule [13].

3.1.4 Input Decimated Ensemble

Input Decimated Ensemble (IDE) is a method for constructing ensembles that selects subsets of features according to their ability to discriminate the classes. In our experiments we use a variant of IDE, proposed in [27], where each classifier is trained using the feature transforms PCA, ICA, and NPE (for details on these transforms, see below in section 3.2) on a subset, randomly extracted, of the training patterns, with each subset containing patterns of only one class.

Outline of Input Decimated Ensemble

Below is a simple pseudocode description of the IDE variant algorithm used in our experiments.

For t = 1, 2, ...T do:

1. Build a random subset $\mathbf{x}_t$ taking randomly selected samples from the original training set;
2. To project the data using the subspace projection w_t calculated using $\mathbf{x}_t$
3. Train a classifier C_t using the training set projected by w_t;
4. Add the classifier to the ensemble.

3.1.5 Rotation Boosting

Rotation Boosting, or RotBoost [40] combines two of the more successful ensemble methods: AdaBoost and Rotation Forest. Both these methods, as noted in section 2, apply a given base learning algorithm to permutated training sets. The only difference in the two methods lies in the way the original training set is perturbed. First a new feature space is obtained by Rotation Forest, then the AdaBoost algorithm is performed on the feature space obtained by Rotation Forest. In our experiments we have used the original source code for RotBoost, which was shared by the authors of [40].

3.1.6 Fuzzy Bagging

Fuzzy Bagging can be considered a supervised version of Bagging, i.e., instead of randomly selecting patterns for a new training set, a supervised selection is performed. This selection is obtained by a Fuzzy C-Means clustering, thereby increasing the diversity among the classifiers that build the ensemble.

Outline of Fuzzy Bagging

Given an original training set S, new training sets, $S_1; \ldots ; S_K$, are generated by partitioning S into K clusters, with set S_i built using the patterns that belong to *i-th* cluster. We assign to a cluster I, 63.2% of the patterns of each class which have the highest membership in that cluster. This value is derived from Bagging, where the probability of being drawn is equally distributed over the training set S. On average, 63.2 is the percentage of training elements contained in each modified training set S_i.

Fuzzy bagging is based on the minimization of the objective function in Eq. 1:

$$J_m = \sum_{i=1}^{m}\sum_{j=1}^{s} u_{ij}^{\alpha}\left\|\mathbf{x}_i - \mathbf{c}_j\right\|^2, \qquad 1 \le \alpha \le \infty \tag{1}$$

where α is any real number greater than 1 (degree of fuzzification), u_{ij} is the degree of membership of $\mathbf{x}_i$ in the cluster j, $\mathbf{x}_i$ is the ith of the m n-dimensional points, $\mathbf{c}_j$ is the center of the cluster j, and ||*|| is the Euclidean distance expressing the similarity between any measured data and the center.

Fuzzy partitioning is the iterative optimization of the objective function of Eq. 1, where the updating equations for the membership u_{ij} and for the cluster centers $\mathbf{c}_j$ are the following:

$$u_{ij} = \frac{1}{\sum_{k=1}^{s}\left(\frac{\left\|\mathbf{x}_i - \mathbf{c}_j\right\|^2}{\left\|\mathbf{x}_i - \mathbf{c}_k\right\|^2}\right)^{\frac{2}{\alpha-1}}} \quad \text{and} \quad \mathbf{c}_j = \frac{\sum_{i=1}^{m} u_{ij}^{\alpha}\mathbf{x}_i}{\sum_{i=1}^{m} u_{ij}^{\alpha}} \tag{2}$$

This procedure converges to a local minimum or a saddle point of $\boldsymbol{J}_m$.

3.1.7 Cluster Selection

Cluster Selection, proposed by [22], tries to create a supervised random subspace for obtaining the new training sets $S_1; \ldots ; S_K$. New training sets are generated by partitioning the original training set into K clusters that separate the training patterns that belong to the same class (i.e., classes are independently partitioned into clusters by Fuzzy C-Means to group together similar patterns), then for each cluster a different feature set is selected for maximizing the discrimination between the cluster and all the other classes. Each new training set, S_i, is given by the concatenation of a cluster with the training patterns of the other classes (where only the features selected for that cluster are retained). In this work we use NPE to reduce the feature space, thus this method could be considered a supervised version of IDE.

3.2 Feature Transforms

In this subsection the feature transform methods used in our experiments are reported and briefly explained.

3.2.1 Principal Component Analysis (PCA)

Principal Component Analysis[2] [6] is the most widely used method for reducing dimensionality. Starting from the covariance matrix of the training patterns, PCA finds a set of eigenvectors and eigenvalues. Dimensionality is reduced by using only those eigenvectors that are most significant.

3.2.2 Independent Component Analysis (ICA)

Independent Component Analysis [12], unlike PCA, which is based on the covariance matrix (i.e., on second order statistics), is based on higher order statistics. ICA computes the reduced basis components that are as statistically independent as possible so that the reduced space is one that minimizes the statistical dependence of the components in the representation.

3.2.3 Neighborhood Preserving Embedding (NPE)

Neighborhood Preserving Embedding was first proposed in [38]. Unlike PCA, which aims at preserving the global Euclidean structure, NPE preserves the local neighborhood structure on the data manifold. Therefore, NPE is less sensitive to outliers than PCA.

The first step in the NPE algorithm is to construct an adjacency graph, where the *i-th* node of the graph corresponds to the *i-th* training pattern $\mathbf{x}_i$. The edge between the nodes i and j is built if $\mathbf{x}_j$ is among the K nearest neighbors of $\mathbf{x}_i$. The weight of the edge from node i to node j is computed by minimizing a given objective function. To compute the linear projections, the generalized eigenvector problem is solved (see [38] for details). The MATLAB code used in our experiments is freely available at http://www.cs.uiuc.edu/homes/dengcai2/Data/data.html.

3.3 Classifier Algorithms

In this subsection we provide a general discussion, followed by an algorithmic outline, of the base classifier used in our ensembles (the decision tree) and of the classifiers used in our stand-alone comparisons.

3.3.1 Decision Trees

A Decision Tree (DT) is a decision support tool in the form of a tree structure. The goal of the tree is to create a model that predicts the value of a target label based on several input features. The advantage of using DT as the base classifier in

---

[2] Implemented as in the PRTools 3.1.7 MATLAB Toolbox.

ensembles is its instability. DT is also simple to understand, works well with hard data, and is easily combined. [39].

Outline of Decision Trees

Each interior node (decision node) corresponds to one of the input features and specifies a test to be carried out on a single feature. The edges to children represent all the possible outcomes of the test of that input feature and indicate the path to be followed. Each leaf node indicates the value of the target label, given the values of the input features represented by the path from the root to the leaf. A tree can be *trained* by splitting the source set into subsets based on testing a single feature. This process is repeated on each derived subset in a recursive manner called *recursive partitioning*. The recursion is completed when the subset of the training patterns at a given node has the same label or when splitting no longer adds value to the predictions. In this work we have used a decision tree with pruning, where the information gain is used as the binary splitting criterion.

3.3.2 Support Vector Machines

Support Vector Machines (SVMs) were first introduced in [37] and are maximum margin classifiers. They are two-class classifiers that find a decision surface that maximizes the distance of the closest points in the training set to the decision boundary.

SVMs use a variety of kernel functions (linear, polynomial, and radial basis functions) as approximating functions. Different types are used depending upon the type of input patterns: a linear maximal margin classifier is used for linearly separable data, a linear soft margin classifier is used for linearly nonseparable, or overlapping, classes, and a nonlinear classifier is used for classes that are overlapped as well as separated by nonlinear hyperplanes. For more information about SVM, the reader is refered to [5].

Outline of SVMs

Linear maximal margin classifier. The goal is to build the hyperplane that maximizes the minimum distance between two classes. This hyperplane has the form:

$$f(\mathbf{x}) = \sum_{i=1}^{k} \alpha_i y_i \mathbf{x}_i \cdot \mathbf{x} + b \tag{3}$$

where α and b are the solutions of a quadratic programming problem.

Unknown test data xt can be classified by simply computing Eq. 4.

$$f(x) = sign(\mathrm{w}_0 \bullet \mathrm{x}_t + b_0) \tag{4}$$

It can be seen by examining the above equation that the hyperplane is determined by all the training data, $\mathbf{x}_i$, that have the corresponding attributes of $\alpha_i > 0$.

Linear soft margin classifier. The goal in this case is to separate the two classes of training data with a minimal number of errors. This is accomplished using non-negative slack variables, $\xi_{i,\ i} = 1, 2, \ldots k$, and a penalty, C, is introduced to control the cost of errors. The computation of the linear soft margin classifier is the same as the linear maximal margin classifier.

Nonlinear classifier. In this case, kernel functions are used to transform the input space to a feature space of higher dimensionality where a linear separating hyperplane that separates the input vectors into two classes can be found. In this case, the hyperplane and decision rule for the nonlinear training pattern is Eq. 5.

$$f(x) = sign(\sum_{i=1}^{K} \alpha_i y_i \quad K(x_t, x) + b). \tag{5}$$

Where, α_i and b are the solutions of a quadratic programming problem and $K(\mathbf{x}_t, \mathbf{x})$ is a kernel function.

3.3.3 Levenberg-Marquardt Neural Networks (LMNN)

The LMNN algorithm [17, 19] is a widely used optimization algorithm that solves the problem of nonlinear least squares minimization using Gauss-Newton's iteration in combination with gradient descent. It is one of the fastest methods for training moderate sized feedforward neural networks. For a more detailed tutorial see [28].

Outline of LMNN

Gradient descent is a simple method for finding the minima in a function. It updates a parameter at each step by adding a negative of the scaled gradient:

$$x_{i+1} = x_i - \lambda \nabla f \tag{6}$$

Eq. 6 can be improved as follows:

$$\nabla f(x) = \nabla f(x_0) + (x - x_0)^T \nabla f(x_0) + \text{higher order terms of } (x - x_0). \tag{7}$$

Ignoring the higher order terms by assuming f to be quadratic around x_0 and solving for the minimum of x by setting the left hand side of Eq. 6 to 0, we obtain Newton's method:

$$x_{i+1} = x_i - (\nabla^2 f(x_i))^{-1} \nabla f(x_i) \ . \tag{8}$$

where x_0 is replaced by x_i and x by x_{i+1}.

LMNN is designed to approach second-order training speed without having to compute the Hessian matrix, which is

$$\mathbf{H} = \mathbf{J}^T\mathbf{J} \, . \tag{9}$$

The gradient can be computed as

$$\mathbf{g} = \mathbf{J}^T\mathbf{e} \, . \tag{10}$$

where **J** is the Jacobian matrix that contains the first derivatives of the network errors with respect to the weights and biases, and **e** is the vector of network errors.

Combining the above equations, Levenberg proposed an algorithm based on Eq. 11:

$$\mathbf{x}_{i+1} = \mathbf{x}_i - [\mathbf{H} + \lambda\mathbf{I}]^{-1}\mathbf{g} \, . \tag{11}$$

Levenberg's algorithm can be outlined as follows:

1. Update weights as in Eq. 11;
2. Evaluate the error of the new parameter vector;
3. If the error has increased, then reset the weights to their previous values and increase λ by a some large factor and goto 1;
4. If the error had decreased, then accept the new values for the weights and decrease λ by a factor a large factor and goto 1.

A problem with the above algorithm is that when λ is large, the Hessian matrix is not used. Marquardt improved the algorithm by replacing the identity matrix in Eq. 9 with the diagonal of the Hessian, resulting the Levenberg-Marquardt update rule:

$$\mathbf{x}_{i+1} = \mathbf{x}_i - [\mathbf{H} + \lambda diag[\mathbf{H}]^{-1}\mathbf{g} \, . \tag{12}$$

By using singular value decomposition (SVD) and other techniques to compute the inverse, the cost of the updates is significantly less than the costs involved in computing the gradient descent for small parameters but eventually the costs become prohibitive when weight size increases.

3.3.4 Gaussian Process Classifier

A Gaussian process is a generalization of the Gaussian probability distribution. A Gaussian Process Classifier (GPC) is a discriminative approach where the class membership probability is the Bernouilli distribution [32]. GPC has a proven track record classifying many different tasks, see [10].

Outline of the Gaussian Transform Classifier

The Gaussian Transform Classifier is based on methods of approximate inference for classification, since the exact inference in Gaussian process models with likelihood functions tailored to classification is intractable. For the rather involved mathematical details of this classification method, the reader would be best served to refer to chapter 3 in [32]. This chapter is electronically available at http://www.gaussian process.org/gpml/. In the experiments in this chapter we have used the code that is available at http://www.gaussianprocess.org/gpml/code/matlab/doc/.

4 Medical Databases

For comparing the proposed approaches with other state-of-the-art approaches, we report results obtained on the following six benchmark datasets available in the UCI Repository:[3]

1. The breast cancer dataset *(BREAST)*
2. The heart disease dataset *(HEART)*
3. The Pima Indians Dataset *(DIAB)*
4. The Wisconsin breast dataset *(WDBC)*
5. A erythemato-squamous disease classification datatset (*DERMA*)
6. A microarray dataset (*Med*)

The BREAST dataset is used to develop better systems to diagnosis breast tumors starting from histopathological features. The HEART dataset is used to predict the presence of heart disease in patients using demographic information along with other measures, such as resting blood pressure and fasting blood sugar. The DIAB dataset is used to forecast the onset of diabetes mellitus. The WDBC dataset, like the BREAST dataset, was developed to diagnosis breasts tumors. The features, however, are computed from a digitized image of a fine needle aspirate of a breast mass. The data describes characteristics of the cell nuclei present in the image.

The erythemato-squamous diseases are psoriasis, seboreic dermatitis, lichen planus, pityriasis rosea, chronic dermatitis, and pityriasis rubra pilaris. These diseases are frequently seen in the outpatient dermatology departments. For the Derma dataset, patients were evaluated clinically on twelve features, and skin samples were taken for the evaluation of 22 histopathological features [9].

The microarray (Med) dataset is used to determine the survival rate of patients with medulloblastomas, the most common malignant brain tumor of childhood. This dataset is composed of 60 samples (patients), with 39 survivors and 21 treatment failures. The data were first normalized by standardizing each column

[3] `http://archive.ics.uci.edu/ml/`

(sample) to a mean of 0 and a standard deviation of 1. Since the dimension of the feature space is very high, only the 60 of the best features are selected, as in [29].

Table 1 summarizes the main characteristics of the datasets in terms of the number of attributes (A), number of examples (E), and the number of classes (C). A detailed description of these databases is available on the UCI machine learning website at http://archive.ics.uci.edu/ml/.

Table 1. Characteristics of the datasets used in the experimentation: A is the number of attributes, E is the number of examples, and C is the number of classes

DATASET	A	E	C
BREAST	9	699	2
HEART	13	303	2
WDBC	30	569	2
PIMA	8	768	2
DERMA[5]	34	358	6
MEDULLO	60	60	2

The evaluation protocol used in our experiments is fairly standard. As suggested by many classification approaches, the features in these datasets are linearly normalized between 0 and 1. Results using these datasets are averaged over ten experiments. For each experiment, except for the MEDULLO and the DERMA datasets, we randomly resample the learning and the testing sets (containing respectively half of the patterns) while maintaining the distribution of the patterns in the classes. For the MEDULLO dataset the *leave-one-out* cross-validation protocol is used, while for the DERMA dataset the 10-fold cross validation method is used. These testing protocol are widely used in the literature for these dataset. The results are reported in terms of error rate.

5 Experimental Results

In this section we compare several classifier ensembles that generalize well. The base classifier, as noted above in section 3.3.1, is the decision tree with pruning,[4] where the information gain is used as the binary splitting criterion.

In Table 2 we reports the performance obtained by the following classifier systems:

- SA, the stand-alone decision tree classifier;
- BAG, a bagging ensemble of 50 classifiers;

---

[4] As implemented as in PrTools 3.1.7
ftp://ftp.ph.tn.tudelft.nl/pub/bob/prtools/prtools3.1.7

- RS, a random subspace ensemble of 50 classifiers;
- FBAG, the fuzzy bagging method;
- Cluster, the Cluster selection method;
- RF-*X*, a Rotation Forest ensemble of 50 classifiers with *M*=3 (as in [27]), where the feature transform *X* is used for building the projection matrix;
- RF-M, a Rotation Forest ensemble, where the ICA feature transform is used for building the projection matrix and the value of the parameter *M* changes between 2 and the number of features divided by 2; these classifiers, where n=[(number of features)/2-2]×T[5], are combined using the Sum Rule.
- RS-X, a random subspace ensemble of 50 X methods;
- FB-X, the fuzzy clustering approach is used for selecting a subset of training pattern in X;
- ID, is the original IDE algorithm, where the PCA transform is used to project the data;
- ID-*X*, is the improved version of IDE, where each class is *partitioned* into several clusters, as in [27]. The feature transform *X* is used for building the projection matrix. The classifiers are combined using the Sum Rule.
- RotB, is the method proposed in [40]; in our experiments 50 classifiers are combined;
- RotB-X, as in RotB, but instead of using only the PCA transform, the feature transform *X* is used for creating the projection matrices.
- SVM, the stand-alone Support Vector Machine; for each dataset, both the kernel and the parameters are optimized for that dataset.
- GPC,[6] the stand-alone Gaussian process classifier [32].
- LMNC, the stand-alone Levenberg-Marquardt neural net classifier.

In table 2, the column *Average* is reporting the average accuracy using the first six datasets.

---

[5] The value of T is chosen for creating 50 classifiers.

[6] The software is available at `http://www.gaussianprocess.org/gpml/`, the parameters are set *loghyper* = [0.0; 2.0].

Table 2. Experimental results of methods on the different datasets

Method	Med	Breast	Heart	Diab	Wdbc	Derma	Average
Sa	35.0	6.9	24	31.7	6.1	3.3	17.8
Bag	26.6	4.9	21.3	24.2	4.6	2.5	14.0
FBag	21.6	4.9	19.2	24.5	5.2	1.9	12.9
Cluster	31.6	3.4	16.8	25.6	5.7	1.6	14.1
RS	26.6	4.3	18.1	26.3	4.5	2.7	13.8
RF-Pca	23.3	4.1	15.7	25.1	2.8	2.2	12.2
RF-Ica	21.6	3.7	15.5	25.1	2.4	1.1	11.6
RF-NPE	23.3	4.0	17.0	25.2	3.1	1.6	12.4
FB-RF-M	21.6	3.5	15.7	23.7	2.6	1.1	11.4
RF-M	21.6	3.5	15.4	24.5	2.4	1.1	11.4
RotB	21.6	3.6	16	25.9	2.8	1.7	11.9
RotB-Ica	21.6	3.9	16.8	25.0	3.1	1.4	12.0
RotB-NPE	18.3	3.0	14.9	25.9	2.5	1.4	11.0
RS-RotBNPE	18.3	3.0	14.6	24.4	2.8	1.4	10.7
ID	30	3.7	24	30.2	5.8	2.7	16.1
ID-PCA	23.3	3.5	16	25.8	3.8	2.7	12.5
ID-Ica	21.6	3.7	17.9	25.3	3.5	3.3	12.5
ID-NPE	25.0	3.5	14.7	24.8	4.1	2.5	12.4
FB-ID	31.6	3.5	16.0	25.6	3.9	2.5	13.9
RS-ID-NPE	23.3	3.1	14.4	24.2	3.3	2.1	11.7
SVM	23.3	3.7	17.3	23.5	3.0	1.9	12.1
GPC	25.0	4.1	16.0	23.3	2.7	1.1	12.0
LMNC	28.3	3.7	20.3	27.6	3.4	5.5	14.8

Analyzing the results reported in Table 2, we can draw the following conclusions:

- The best performing ensemble methods are RotB-NPE and RF-M. They outperform not only the other ensemble methods using decision trees but also SVM. RS and SVM outperform GPC, RotB-NPE, and RF-M.
- None of the tested feature transforms generalizes better than any of the others, i.e., none outperforms any of the others across all the datasets.
- Ensemble methods based on feature transforms outperform other ensemble methods on all the datasets
- GPC obtains a performance that is similar to SVM,

- A very interesting result is obtained in the DERMA dataset, where an error rate of 1.1% is lower than the best previously published result [36].
- It is very interesting to note that RS ensembles are shown to be quite useful; the RS-ID-NPE outperforms ID-NPE, and the RS-RotB-NPE outperforms Rot B-NPE.

Table 3. Performance obtained by SVM, LMNC and GPC

Method		Med	Breast	Heart	Diab	Wdbc	Derma	Average
SVM	Sa	23.3	3.7	17.3	23.5	3.0	1.9	12.1
	Bagging	28.3	3.3	16.3	23.5	3.3	12.5	14.5
	RandS	23.3	3.7	13.9	24.7	3.8	5.2	12.4
LMNC	Sa	28.3	3.7	20.3	27.6	3.4	5.5	14.8
	Bagging	26.6	3.7	16.0	24.3	3.0	1.9	12.6
	RandS	26.6	3.3	15.5	24.1	3.0	4.1	12.7
	BEST ensemble	28.3	4.6	18.0	27.0	3.5	1.4	13.8
GPC	Sa	25.0	4.1	16.0	23.3	2.7	1.1	12.0
	Bagging	23.3	3.8	16.0	23.4	2.4	1.3	11.7
	RandS	23.3	3.9	13.6	23.5	2.3	1.1	11.2

In Table 3 we report the performance obtained by three stand-alone classifiers (SVM, LMNC, GPC) and their bagging versions (BAG), random subspace versions (RS) and RotB-NPE (where only the LMNC classifier is used, since SVM and GPC are not well suited for building RotB-NPE ensembles).

In these experiments it is interesting to note that only LMNC ensembles are useful, and again the older RS methods outperform a RotB-NPE using LMNC. It is probably for this reason that recent ensembles proposed and studied in the literature are primarily based on decision trees. For GPC classifiers, RS only slightly outperforms the stand-alone approach.

4 Conclusion

In this chapter, we make an extensive study of artificial intelligence (AI) techniques that can be used in data mining the stockpiles of databases in healthcare.

The goal of this paper is to discover methods for building a generalized ensemble of classifiers that will perform well across a host of medical problems. We performed an empirical comparison between several ensemble methods and classifier systems using eight databases that address very different medical problems and that combine multiple sources of data. Our experimental results show that novel ensembles of decision trees outperform SVM in several datasets. Furthermore, the experimental results show our ensemble methods obtain an error reduction that is equal to if not greater than the best performing systems published in the literature.

Unfortunately, it was not possible for us to find a single ensemble method, i.e., a general purpose ensemble, that outperformed all the other classifiers across all eight tested datasets. Nonetheless, some interesting findings are reported.

We conclude by noting how machine learning technologies can augment medical diagnosis. Machine learning methods offer great flexibility in modeling problems and reasonable accuracy in prediction, as compared with human experts. Moreover, it is easy for machine learning technologies to combine data from multiple sources into one system. This increases the potential for discovering hidden patterns in the data and eventually better healthcare outcomes.

Acknowledgements

The authors would like to thank C-X. Zhang and J-S. Zhang for sharing their Matlab code of RotBoost.

References

1. Alpaydin, E.: Introduction to machine learning. MIT Press, Cambridge, MA (2004)
2. Bologna, G., Appel, R.D.: A comparison study on protein fold recognition. In: The 9th Int Conference on Neural Information Processing, Singapore, pp. 2492–2496 (2002)
3. Breiman, L.: Bagging predictors 24(2), 123–140 (1996)
4. Breiman, L.: Random forest 45(1), 5–32 (2001)
5. Cristianini, N., Shawe-Taylor, J.: An introduction to support vector machines and other kernel-based learning methods. Cambridge University Press, Cambridge, UK (2000)
6. Duda, R.O., Hart, P.E., Stork, D.G.: Pattern classification. Wiley, New York (2000)
7. Freund, Y., Schapire, R.E.: A decision-theoretic generalization of on-line learning and an application to boosting. J. Comput. Syst. Sci. 55(1), 119–139 (1997)
8. Guo, J., Lin, Y.: Tssub: Eukaryotic protein subcellar localization by extracting features from profiles 22, 1784–1785 (2006)
9. Güvenir, H.A., Demiröz, G., Iter, N.: Learning differential diagnosis of erythemato-squamous diseases using voting feature intervals 13, 147–165 (1998)
10. Han, D., Bo, L., Sminchisescu, C.: Selection and context for action recognition, Xian, China (2009)
11. Ho, T.K.: The random subspace method for constructing decision forests 20(8), 832–844 (1998)
12. Hyvärinen, A.: The fixed-point algorithm and miximum likelihood estimation for independent component analysis 10, 1–5 (1999)

13. Kittler, J.: On combining classifiers 20(3), 226–239 (1998)
14. Kuncheva, L.I.: Combining pattern classifiers: Methods and algorithms. Wiley, New York (2004)
15. Kuncheva, L.I., Whitaker, C.J.: Measures of diversity in classifier ensembles and their relationship with the ensemble accuracy 51(2), 181–207 (2003)
16. Lan, H., Carson, R., Provart, N., Bonner, A.: Combining classifiers to predict gene function in arabidopsis thaliana using large-scale gene expression measurements 8, 358 (2007)
17. Levenberg, K.: A method for the solution of certain nonlinear problems in least squares. Quart Appl. Math. 2(2), 164–168 (1944)
18. Liu, K., Huang, D.: Cancer classification using rotation forest 38(5), 601–610 (2008)
19. Marquardt, D.: An algorithm for least-squares estimation of nonlinear parameters 11, 431–441 (1963)
20. Martínez-Muñoz, G., Suárez, A.: Switching class labels to generate classification ensembles 38(10), 1483–1494 (2005)
21. Melville, P., Mooney, R.J.: Creating diversity in ensembles using artificial, information fusion 6(1), 99–111 (2005)
22. Nanni, L.: Cluster-based pattern discrimination: A novel technique for feature selection 27(6), 682–687 (2006)
23. Nanni, L., Lumini, A.: Fuzzybagging: A novel ensemble of classifiers 39(3), 488–490 (2006)
24. Nanni, L., Lumini, A.: Mpps: An ensemble of support vector machines based on multiple physicochemical properties of amino-acids 69(13), 1688–1690 (2006)
25. Nanni, L., Lumini, A.: Ensemblator: An ensemble of classifiers for reliable classification of biological data 28(5), 622–630 (2007)
26. Nanni, L., Lumini, A.: Ensemble generation and feature selection for the identification of students with learning disabilities (accepted 2008)
27. Nanni, L., Lumini, A.: Using ensemble of classifiers in bioinformatics. In: Nanni, L., Lumini, A. (eds.) Machine learning research progress, Nova publishers, New York (2008) (accepted)
28. Nocedal, J., Wright, S.J.: Numerical optimization. Springer, New York (1999)
29. Pomeroy, S.L., Tamayo, P., Gaasenbeek, M., Sturla, L.M., Angelo, M., McLaughlin, M.E., Kim, J.Y.H., Goumnerova, L.C., Black, P.M., Lau, C., Allen, J.C., Zagzag, D., Olson, J.M., Curran, T., Wetmore, C., Biegel, J.A., Poggio, T., Mukherjee, S., Rifkin, R., Califano, A., Stolovitzky, G., Louis, D.N., Mesirov, J.P., Lander, E.S., Golub, T.R.: Prediction of central nervous system embryonal tumour outcome based on gene expression 415(1), 436–442 (2002)
30. Pudil, P., Novovicova, J., Kittler, J.: Floating search methods in feature selection. Pattern Recognition Letters 5(11), 1119–1125 (1994)
31. Ranawana, R., Palade, V.: A neural network based multiclassifier system for gene identification in DNA sequences 14, 122–131 (2005)
32. Rasmussen, C.E., Williams, K.I.: Gaussian processes for machine learning. The MIT Press, Cambridge, MA (2006)
33. Rodriguez, J.J., Kuncheva, L.I., Alonso, C.J.: Rotation forest: A new classifier ensemble method 28(10), 1619–1630 (2006)
34. Russell, S., Norvig, P.: Artificial intelligence: A modern approach. Prentice Hall, Upper Saddle River, NJ (2002)

35. Tumer, K., Oza, N.C.: Input decimated ensembles 6, 65–77 (2003)
36. Übeyli, E.D.: Combined neural networks for diagnosis of erythemato-squamous diseases (2008), doi:10.1016/j.eswa.2008.06.002
37. Vapnik, V.N.: The nature of statistical learning theory. Springer, New York (1995)
38. Xiaofei, H., Cai, D., Yan, S., Zhang, H.-J.: Neighborhood preserving embedding. In: Tenth IEEE International Conference on Computer Vision (ICCV 2005), Beijing, China (2005)
39. Yuan, Y., Shaw, M.J.: Introduction to fuzzy decision trees 69, 125–139 (1995)
40. Zhang, C.-X., Zhang, J.-S.: Rotboost: A technique for combining rotation forest and adaboost 29(10), 1524–1536 (2008)

Chapter 5
Medical Diagnosis Decision Support HMAS under Uncertainty HMDSuU

Israa Al-Qaysi[1], Rainer Unland[1], Claus Weihs[2], and Cherif Branki[3]

[1] Institute for Computer Science and Business Information Systems
University of Duisburg-Essen 45117 Essen, Germany
{israa.al-qaysi,rainer.unland}@icb.uni-due.de
http://www.dawis.wiwi.uni-due.de/team/esra-al-kaysi/
http://www.dawis.wiwi.uni-due.de/team/rainer-unland/

[2] Dortmund University, Department of Statistics
44221 Dortmund, Germany
weihs@statistik.uni-dortmund.de
http://www.statistik.tu-dortmund.de/weihs.html

[3] University of the West of Scotland, Paisley Scotland
Cherif.Branki@uws.ac.uk
www.uws.ac.uk

Abstract. Fast, reliable, and correct medical diagnostics is of utter importance in today's world where diseases can spread quickly. For this reason, we have developed a medical diagnosis system that is based on multi agent system theory, the holonic paradigm, and swarm intelligence techniques. More specifically, a huge number of comparatively simple agents form the basis of our system. In order to provide a solid medical diagnosis always a set of relevant agents needs to work together. These agents will provide a huge set of possible solutions, which need to be evaluated in order to conclude. The paradigm of swarm intelligence implies that a set of comparatively simple entities produces sophisticated and highly reliable results. In our scenario, it means that our agents are not provided with a real world model; i.e., it has only a very limited understanding on health issues and the process of medical diagnosis. This puts a huge burden on the decision process.

This paper concentrate on the decision process within our system and will present our ideas, which are based on decision theory, and here, especially, on Bayesian probability since, among others, uncertainty is inherent feature of a medical diagnosis process. The presented approach focuses on reaching the optimal medical diagnosis with the minimum risk under the given uncertainty. Additional factors that play an important role are the required time for the decision process and the produced costs.

Keywords: Multi agent system, holonic, self-organization, emergence, swarm intelligence, stigmergy, decision theory, uncertainty, bayesian probability.

S. Brahnam & L.C. Jain (Eds.): Adv. Comput. Intell. Paradigms in Healthcare 5, SCI 326, pp. 67–94.
springerlink.com

1 Introduction

Medical practitioners encounter several difficulties throughout the ability of diagnosis decision making for patients. The cause of these difficulties is the uncertainty situation in the nature of health information. From this point, there is a need to consolidate medical diagnosis decision throughout computerized diagnostic decision support systems, where recently, the process of medical diagnosis is becoming increasingly computerized. Moreover, Bayes probability expected risk, and optimal decision with the total risk is the essential aspects of decision analysis.

Primarily, uncertainty is often a central aspect of medicine in general [Jerzy 91] [Conrad 76]. It comes from the limits of medical knowledge, which is a mixture of scientifically precise and clinical impressions leaving much space for medical uncertainty. In particular, uncertainty is often an important factor in medical diagnosis. In fact, the symptoms that the patient has could be a symbol of any one of a number of illnesses or may be no illness at all. Uncertainty is a core element of modern medicine where diagnosis is the classification of medical knowledge in disease categories. Uncertainty appears because there may be overlaps among diverse areas of diseases. Furthermore, may be a patient suffers from a mixture of diseases, the unknown one.

Medical diagnosis decision support holonic multi agent system is particularly helpful in that. It is able to improve the accessibility of knowledge of patient symptoms, consequential in quality improvement of the diagnostic process and increase of efficiency, and then reduces costs. Furthermore, decision theory helps decision maker to make an optimal medical diagnosis together with swarm techniques and holonic paradigm.

According to the requirements of individual autonomy and social interaction ability of agent, the mechanism of how to constitute simple agents and intelligence was studied by combining holonic multi agent system and swarm intelligence techniques on the premise of autonomy.

This paper is organized as follows: the next section discusses the state of the art. Section 3 introduces basic concepts starting with holonic organizations with multi agent system. Section 4 presents the decision theory with the decision under uncertainty. In section 5, we describe our unification of the Holonic Medical Diagnostic System (HMDSuU) Under Uncertainty framework. Finally, section 6 concludes the paper.

2 State of the Art

There are many areas in the Medical domain covering different direction that would take advantage from health care system with all its aspects. Health care systems are complex; recent years have shown a shift in focus in health care domain. The core of medical problems is the diagnosis approach, which is the process of identifying a medical state or disease by its symptoms, signs, and from the results of different diagnostic procedures. Many medical diagnosis systems are proposed in the medical domain.

Medical diagnosis support system with neural networks has been proposed. Signs, symptoms, remarks, clinical laboratory data such as blood and biochemical check up data, are fundamental information. The system identification algorithm has also been used to compare the weighted value using patient information with relevant sample based on medical knowledge [Matsumoto 04].

Computer supported cooperative work (CSCW) has been reported ([Lu 05], [Lu 06], [Lu 05a]) provides a dynamic environment for oral medical professionals to access patient information and enhances the capacities of the patient consultation, medical record management and interactive medical service.

Four different kinds of classifiers, namely, Bayesian, k-NN, k-Means and 2-D SOM have been used to classify the thyroid gland data set. The performance of classification algorithms on the diagnosis of thyroid dysfunctional visualized them in the form of multi-class extension of ROC analysis [Banu 08].

Probability [Stensmo 96] models are constructed using mixture models that are efficiently learned by the Expectation-Maximization algorithm. Problems with missing data are then solved. Decision theory is used to find the most informative. Clinical decision support system was proposed by Catley ([Catley 03], [Catley 03a], [Yang 04], [Catley 2004], and [Catley 04a]) to diagnose babies in neonatal intensive case unit and assess the effectiveness of real-time decision support. CDSSs using the eXtended Markup Language (XML) and it is subsequently offered as a secure web service.

Like the previous systems that work in isolation, it cannot overcome the potential of diagnosis for complex process. Some of these drawbacks have been solved with expert systems. Medical Expert systems are able to motive with data from patients to come up with a reasonable conclusions. Expert systems can be applied in various areas of medical domains like diagnostic assistance, agents for information retrieval, expert laboratory information systems and generating alerts and reminders...etc.

DXplain ([Barnett 98], [Elhanan 96], [Barnett 96], [Banu 08], [Feldman 91], and [Barnett 1987]) is a Clinical decision support expert system that can be used as a medical reference system, as a diagnostic clinical decision support tool, and as an electronic medical textbook. It is also available in the World Wide Web. The system uses an interactive format to collect clinical information to produce a ranked list of diagnoses that may be associated with at least some of the clinical manifestations.

Quick Medical Reference (QMR) is a decision support system specified diagnostic data about more than 600 medical diseases. The authors investigated how frequently the correct diagnosis would come out among the five highest ranked diagnoses generated by QMR ([Lemaire 99], [Mabry 91]) that helps physicians to diagnose adult diseases. QMR was designed for three types of use: as an electronic textbook, as an expert consultant program, as an intermediate level spreadsheet for the combination and exploration of simple diagnostic concepts.

Mycin [Shortliffe 76] is an early expert system and it is one of the best-known expert systems to help doctors in antimicrobial drugs to prescribe such drugs for blood infections. In other words, Mycin is a program for advising physicians on treating bacterial infections of the blood and meningitis.

Milho [Milho 00] has presented a web supported development tool specific for medical diagnosis, which is based on Bayesian networks. The proposed system provides a user-friendly interface, giving the users (experts in the medical domain) the possibility to design diagnostic applications without deep background knowledge on Bayesian networks theory.

PUFF [Aikens 83] is a Pulmonary Function System; it is also one of the few expert systems, which has become a helpful tool in its domain of expertise. PUFF is a small expert system, which contains about 400 rules and 75 clinical parameters. The expert system generates information from a set of interpretation statements for pulmonary function diagnosis.

The Causal ASsociational NETworks (CASNET /Glaucoma) is a general tool for building expert system for the conclusion and treatment of diseases (glaucoma), which consists of strategies of decision-making [Kulikowski 82]. Expert clinical knowledge was proposed in a causal-associational network model.

MYCIN, PUFF, QMR, DXplain, and other systems have some problems that are related to expert systems, represented by the difficulties to solve the complexities of medical diagnosis. In other words, medical diagnosis needs more aspects like increased autonomy in process, capability of communication and cooperation with other systems. In fact, agents contain these proprieties. Expert system agent arises afterward to cover the needs of the diagnosis. Moreover, multi agent systems are more flexible, extensible, and adaptable. The expert system agents can cooperate with other agents and humans during the problems solving.

CMDS ([Iantovics 07], [Iantovics 06]) is a hybrid system with human and artificial agents. Expert system agents have been described that it based on the blackboard problem solving with a set of agents. Every agent of the CMDS system has problems solving capability and capacity. The capacity of an agent consists in the quantity of problems that can be solved by the agent, using the existent problem solving resources. During its operation, a medical agent may require the help of assistant agents. Each human and artificial medical agent knows at least one assistant agent whose help may be required. If it is necessary, an assistant agent may cooperate with other assistant agents.

Multi Agent Systems ([Yang 08], [Shieh 08]) have been proposed in several different kinds of problems in the health care area. A multi agent diagnosis helping system (MADHS) is considered as cooperative agents in medical diagnosis. Coordinator, Joint Decision Maker, Examiners, and Specialists are the types of the agent classes that appeared in MADHS. In this paper, organizational structuring is applied in MADHS in order to facilitate the cooperation among agents. Fuzzy Decision Tree collective with certainty factor calculation has been proposed to deal with fuzziness and uncertainty.

Agent-Based Applications [Moreno 03] have been proposed in a Medical Decision Support System with the Diabetes Trials of Oxford University.

Hudson and Cohen have described an IDSS [Hudson 02] to assist in the identification of cardiac diseases. The system uses five agents plus the medical professional to evaluate factors in congestive heart failure, including the use of output from one agent as input to another. Agent can monitor patient conditions, supply information to the physician over the Internet.

Magnetic Resonance Spectroscopy (MRS), HR-MASand, and MRS are three techniques that have been addressed in Health Agents multi-layer framework through multi agent decision support over a distributed network of local databases or Data Marts for Brain Tumour Diagnosis [Arus 06].

Holonic Multi agent System (HMAS) is much more self-organizing and flexible in view of the fact that the holons are self-reliant units that have a degree of autonomy to make its own decision on their exacting level of existence without asking higher-level holons for support. In fact, an open issue of HMAS is to give holons means of self-organization to satisfy their goals. A Holon is a self-similar structure composed of holons as sub-structures. This hierarchical structure composed of holons is called a holarchy. It has two aspects, from one side; Holon is a whole-part construct that is composed of other holons, excluding it is, at the same time, a component of a higher-level holon. A more detailed description can be found in [Koestler 67]. Holonic MAS is an innovative technology designed to support the development of complex, distributed, and heterogeneous information systems.

Diagnostic problems need high quality aspects to solve in the health care. [Ulieru 00, 02, 03, 03a, 03b, 06] suggest the proposal of Internet-enabled Soft Computing Holarchies for e-Health Applications. Their approach builds on remote access to patient information for multifactor decision making in case of emergency. Representing holons as software agents enables the development of e-Health environments as web-centric medical holarchies with a wide area of application in tele-medicine.

Holonic medical diagnosis system (HMDSuU) has been organized according to the principles of swarm intelligence. This system combines the advantages of the holonic paradigm, multi agent system technology, neural networks, and swarm intelligence in order to realize a highly reliable, adaptive, scalable, flexible, and robust Internet-based diagnosis system for diseases.

A good overview about the expert systems of medical domains and multi agent systems can also be found in ([Moreno 03], [Bravata 04], and [Foster 05]).

3 Basic Concepts

3.1 Medical Diagnosis and Its Process

In medicine, diagnosis is a very complex process, by which a doctor searches for the disease that best explains the symptoms of a patient. The term "diagnostic criteria" designates the combination of signs, symptoms, and test results that allows the manager or consultant to ascertain the diagnosis of the respective disease or malfunction within the organization. Typically, someone with abnormal symptoms will consult a physician, who will then obtain a history of the patient's illness and examine him for signs of disease. The physician will formulate a hypothesis of probable diagnoses and, in many cases, will obtain further testing to confirm or clarify the diagnosis before providing treatment; in other word,

Identification of disease and treatment proposal based on provided patient's data. The process that may continue in a number of iterations in anticipation of the patient is finally diagnosed with enough certainty and the cause of the symptoms is recognized [Wikipedia, Kappen 02].

The use of computer programs in the diagnostic process has been a protracted term goal of research in information technology and; definitely, it is the most typical application of artificial intelligence and may be one of the particular characteristics of both medical knowledge and the diagnostic task. An accurate diagnosis will, in most cases, lead to suitable treatment.

3.2 Agent and Multi Agent Systems

An agent is a collection of a small amount of features in software capable to solve complex problems. Agents do not simply act in response to their environment. Agents are able to exhibit purposive behavior and performance by taking the initiative, which means that an agent is Proactive. Agents can be competent of flexible and autonomous in environment to convene its design objectives. Technically, agents have roles, behaviors, functionalities, and goals. An agent makes a decision about what action to perform based on the history of the system that it has witnessed to date.

Actually, if each agent is connected; after that, everything has to be a part of a particular system. In addition, if each agent has to take decisions on its own with its capacity, then such a system is a Multi agent system (MAS).

A system is a pair containing an agent and an environment: to create a system that is pervasively embedded in the environment, completely connected, intuitive, portable, and constantly available. Each node of the system should be able to initiate its tasks and actions based on what it learned, with its interaction with other nodes.

An agent may enjoy several fundamental concepts in various combinations. These properties include:

- *Autonomy:* Autonomy refers to the principle that agents manage without the intervention of external elements. In particular, agents decide for themselves whether or not to perform an action.
- *Social:* The ability to act together with other agents or humans by way of variety of agent communication language and works towards common goals.
- *Reactivity:* Maintains a current interaction with its environment.
- *Adaptability:* Agents are characterized via their flexibility, facility, and adaptation to achieve their own goals based on their inherent intention.

- *Learning:* Agent progress performance and quality over time Since Agents learn via their experience.
- *Pro-activity:* Pro-activeness refers to the agent's ability to get the initiative rather than acting simply in response to their environment, generate and attempt to achieve goals.

3.3 Holonic Multi Agent System

Many years ago, Arthur Koestler proposed the word "holon" in "The Ghost in the Machine" [Koestler 67]. It is a combination from the Greek holos = whole, with the suffix "on" which, as in proton or neutron, suggests a particle or part. Arthur Koestler said that all organisms are holons, which are characterized by differentiation, cooperation, and boundaries. A cell is a Holon. Multi agent system is used to solve problems that are too large, to provide a solution to inherently distributed problems and increased reliability.

Holons are self-reliant units that have a degree of autonomy to make its own decision on their exacting level of existence without asking higher-level holons for support. In fact, an open issue of HMAS is to give holons means of self-organization to satisfy their goals. A Holon is a self-similar structure composed of holons as sub-structures. This hierarchical structure composed of holons is called a holarchy. It has two aspects, from one side; Holon is a whole-part construct that is composed of other holons, excluding it is, at the same time, a component of a higher-level Holon. A more detailed description can be found in [Koestler 07].

3.4 Self-organization and Emergence

The connection between emergence and self-organization remains a research question. A self-organizing system is a system, which changes its essential structure as a function of its experience and environment [Koestler 07].

Properly defined, however, any system is called self-organizing if it is able to determine its inner structure by itself as the environment changes. Holonic self-organization combines one of the important aspects of hierarchical and hierarchical organizational structures by clustering the entities of the system into nested hierarchies [DIL91]. The perception of self-organization is central to the explanation of biological systems and software agents that are inherently self-organized.

Occasionally, the perception of self-organization is conflated with that of the correlated concept of emergence. Emergence is a fundamental attribute of process; it would be difficult and complex without the process of emergence. From other side, the emergent behavior is also hard due to the number of communications between each of the components increases combinatorial of a system with the new components and subtle types of behavior to emerge. Emergent property could come into view when a number of agents are activated in an environment.

3.5 Swarm Intelligence and Stigmergy

Swarm Intelligence (SI) is an Artificial Intelligence technique whereby the collective behaviors of simple agents interacting locally with each other, directly or indirectly, and with their environment causing coherent functional global patterns to emerge. SI distributed a problem solving not including centralized control. In other words, SI coordinates each other without need for any communication. The initiative of Swarm Intelligence focuses on the ant search foraging behavior as a metaphor for distributed problem solving.

We metaphor the idea from the ant colonies to be very close to our system where ants communicate with each other by using chemical substances known as pheromones. Ants place smells. After that, ants, which reinforce the trail with food to the colony, follow this pheromone trail. When the food source is exhausted, then no new trails are marked by returning ants and the scent slowly dissipates [Klüver 03].

Ants need this behavior to adapt with changes in the environment. A holonic system could be compared with the ant colony so that each ant is a holon to finding a shorter path, and leaving an suitable pheromone for other ants to follow this trial; an ant colony has a higher capability resulting and quality that cooperate and adapt to changing circumstances with its environment from the collective intelligence of individual ants.

Stigmergy is a key aspect of swarm intelligence and it is a form of self-organization. The idea of stigmergy was introduced by Pierre-Paul Grasse in the 1950's to illustrate the indirect contact happening between individuals in insect societies. It occurs through modifications brought by the individual components to their local environment. Stigmergy produces complex, intelligent structures without Advance planning and supports which have efficient collaboration among simple agents.

Swarm intelligence and stigmergy technique will fully enhance the system although the simplicity of the constituent elements of system. Through the addition of some important features required for the purposes of obtaining the optimal medical diagnosis decision, which, in turn, requires quality attributes like flexibility, adaptability, and robustness.

4 Decision Theory

Decision theory is an organization of knowledge and related analytical techniques of different degrees of procedure, designed to assist a decision maker chosen among a set of alternatives in light of their possible consequences [Frederick 05]. Decision theory can be relevant to conditions of certainty, risk, or uncertainty and seeks to find strategies that maximize the expected value of a utility function which measures the desirability of possible outcomes.

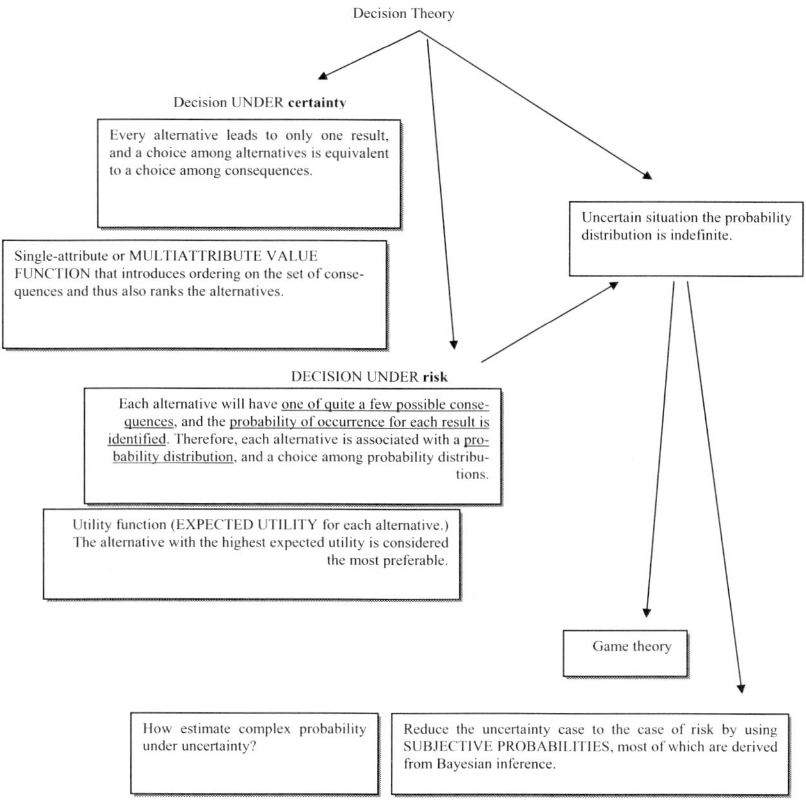

Bayesian decision making is making a decision about the state of nature based on how probable that state is.

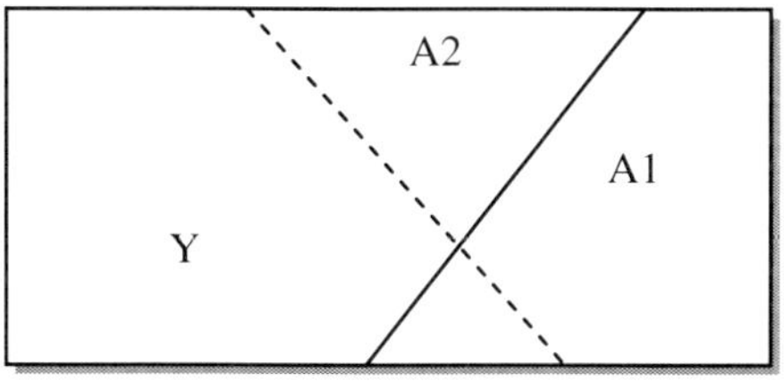

With Bayesian decision making, it would be achievable to settle on the probability that Y belongs to either A1 or A2. Although in the above example, it is obvious that Y is more likely to belong to A2 than A1, the answer is usually not as clear. In other words, Bayesian decision theory helps to examine options to provide an order and provide alternative means of organizing potential [Charles 04].

Decision Medical diagnosis quality is an important point for human beings, and from other side, it is complicated task, but with holonic multi agent system and swarm intelligent technology, it would be a challenge and very useful. In this paper, we worked to contrast the broad aspect of quality. Importance of accurate medical diagnosis was the focus of this work. From one side and from this point the reason for the limited data used in some cases, our work focus on the integration of accurate information in the system with the input data used for the purpose of obtaining diagnostic accuracy. From the other side, it is to show how to decide the optimal medical diagnosis with the minimum risk. Moreover, for this purpose, reducing each of time and cost will be another intention. In other words, Bayesian decision-making provides opportunities to solve the problem of uncertain medical diagnosis decision.

4.1 Decision-Making under Uncertainty

Optimal decisions of medical diagnosis can be obtained using Bayesian decision theory. Such decisions are based on the Bayesian theorem under uncertainty enabling the quantity of the probability of an occurrence based on a prior estimate of its probability and new interpretation. In other words, the Bayesian decision updates its beliefs on the incident of an event based on new information [Timothy 04].

Bayesian decision making is making a decision about the state of nature based on how probable that state is. The elements of Bayesian decision making include the following behaviors:

1) The decision will be taken from a set of appropriate possible states of nature.

$$W = \{\omega_1, \omega_2, \ldots\ldots, \omega_m\} \quad .$$

2) Set up a prior probability in the region of [0,1] which is a prior belief according to the state of nature in which

$$\mathrm{P}(W) = \sum_{i=1}^{m} P(\omega_i) = 1 \quad .$$

3) Denote each of probable actions

$$\mathrm{A} = \{a_1, a_2, \ldots\ldots a_n\} \quad .$$

4) Now assume the following cost (loss) metric

$\lambda_{i,j} =$

	ω_1	ω_2......	ω_m
a_1			
a_2....			
a_n			

5) Considering an expected risk or central estimate of risk

$$R(a_i) = \sum_{j=1}^{m} P(\omega_j)\lambda_{i,j} \quad .$$

This step could be the last one and choose the minimum expected risk action.

6) We can do more to be more certain through calculate class conditional probabilities then to calculate conditional risk given the following observation

$$X_k = \{x_1, x_2, \ldots\ldots, x_r\}.$$

$$R(a_i \mid x_k) = \sum_{\omega j} p(\omega_j \mid x_k) \cdot \lambda_{i,j} \quad .$$

$$P(\omega_j \mid x) = \frac{P(x_k \mid \omega_j).P(\omega_j)}{P(x_k)} \quad .$$

That means

$$posterior = \frac{likelihood \times prior}{evidence} \quad .$$

$$P(x_k) = \sum_{j=1}^{m} P(x_k \mid \omega_j).P(\omega_j) \quad .$$

On the other hand, Class conditional probabilities provides a solution to the problem of how to learn from new data

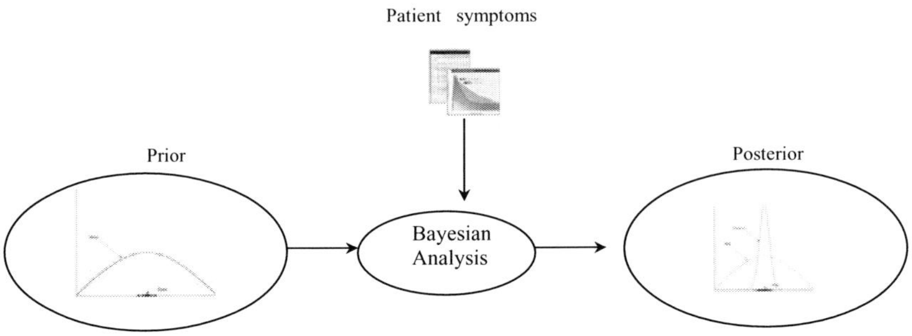

Fig. 2. Bayesian analysis

Prior probability distribution, or, simply, the prior of an uncertain quantity, is the probability distribution that express the uncertainty about the probability before the data are taken into account [James 85]. In fact, for more input data, we will get a lower probability of error.

Properly, the probability of error is:

$$\mathbf{P}(\text{error}|\mathbf{x}) = \begin{cases} P(\omega_1|x) & \textit{if} \text{ we decide } \omega_2 \\ P(\omega_2|x) & \textit{if} \text{ we decide } \omega_1 \end{cases}$$

Consequently, deciding on the status that has the higher posterior probability minimizes the probability of error.

4.2 Optimal Bayesian Decision

The total risk of a decision function is given by

$$E_{p(x)}[R(\alpha(x)\mid x)] = \sum_{x} p(x)\cdot R(\alpha(x)\mid x) .$$

A decision function is optimal if it minimizes the total risk. This optimal total risk is called Bayesian risk.

4.3 General Equation of Bayes' Rule for the Symptom Complex

I have tried to provide as simple an explanation as possible of how the general equation of Bayes' rule for the symptom complex can be arrived at by following the steps in the derivation.

Additionally, mathematically, dividing the number of cases of disease in a population at a given time $n(D)$ by the number of people in that population N then we will get the probability of disease:

$$P(D)=\frac{n(D)}{N}.$$

In the same way, the probability of a symptom can be written:

$$P(S)=\frac{n(S)}{N}.$$

The probability of symptoms in a given disease can be articulated as:

$$P(S/D)=\frac{n(SD)}{n(D)}.$$

Where $n(SD)$ is the number of patients having both the disease and the symptom in the same time and $n(D)$ is the total number of patients, which have certain disease.

The previous equation could be inversely positioned to the next function:

$$P(D/S)=\frac{n(SD)}{n(S)}.$$

What is the probability of disease occurring when symptoms obtains?

Afterwards, dividing the right-hand side on N as follows:

$$P(D/S)=\frac{n(SD)/N}{n(S)/N}.$$

While $n(SD)/N$ is the probability of both symptoms and diseases and $n(S)/N$ is the probability of symptoms, in that case:

$$P(D/S)=\frac{P(SD)}{p(S)}. \tag{1}$$

Through the same formula, the probability of symptoms in a given disease will be:

$$P(S/D)=\frac{P(SD)}{p(D)}. \qquad (2)$$

From 1, 2

$$P(D)P(S/D)=P(S)P(D/S).$$

Then

$$P(D/S)=\frac{P(D)P(S/D)}{P(S)}. \qquad (3)$$

Since $P(D/S)$ is the simplest form of Bayes' rule, which is the probability of having disease for given symptoms. $P(D)$ is the probability of disease in the population. $P(S)$ is the probability of symptoms in the population, but this formula is not correct for more than one symptoms.

The next steps will be very significant for the purpose of developing simple Bayes' formula to contract in the company of sets for symptoms and diseases. Equally important, the probability of symptoms has to be more clarified where $P(S)$ represents the entire prevalence of the symptom in the population with and without the disease in the population. Then, isolating the symptoms, which are without disease D_1, for instance, into other diseases like $D_2, D_3,...D_k$.

$$n(S)=\sum_{i=1}^{k} n(SD_i) \quad .$$

divided by N

$$n(S)/N=\sum_{i=1}^{k} n(SD_i)/N \quad .$$

At the same time, $n(SD)/N$ is the probability of jointly symptoms and diseases after that

$$P(S)=\sum_{i=1}^{k} P(SD_i) \quad .$$

The symptom and the diseases are found together in the population.

whereas:

$$P(S/D)=\frac{P(SD_i)}{p(D_i)} \Rightarrow$$

$$P(SD_i)=P(D_i)P(S/D_i).$$

Then:

$$P(S)=\sum_{i=1}^{k}P(D_i)P(S/D_i).$$

Probability of having symptoms if disease $D_1 or D_2 or ..., D_K$ is present.

For symptoms complex $S_1, S_2, ..., S_j$ which are to be included for assessment.

$$P(D_i|(S_1,S_2,...S_j)=\frac{P(D_i)P((S_1,S_2,...S_j)|D_i)}{P(S_1,S_2,...S_j)}. \quad (4)$$

If it is assumed that, the Di's are mutually exclusive, then:

$$P(S_1,S_2,...S_j)=\sum_{j=1}^{k}P((S_1,S_2,...S_j)|D_j)P(D_j) \quad .$$

Therefore, that eqn. (4) takes the following form:

$$P(D_i|(S_1,S_2,...S_j)=\frac{P(D_i)P((S_1,S_2,...S_j)|D_i)}{\sum_{j=1}^{k}P((S_1,S_2,...S_j)|D_j)P(D_j)}. \quad (5)$$

From eqn. (5), we can derive two eqns. depending on the relation among symptoms if and only if the symptoms $S_1, S_2, ..., S_j$ are independent of each others, then

$$P(S)=P(S_1)P(S2)...P(S_j) \quad .$$

$$P((S_1,S_2,...S_j)|D_i)=P(S_1|D_i)P(S_2|D_i)P(S_3|D_i)....P(S_n|D_i).$$

$$P(D_i/S_1,S_2,...S_j)=\frac{P(D_i)P(S_1/D_i)...P(S_j/D_i)}{\sum_{i=1}^{k}P(D_i)P(S_1/D_i)...P(S_j/D_i)} \quad (6)$$

The complete Bayes' formula is for the complex independent symptoms $S_1, S_2, ..., S_j$ and set of mutually exclusive diseases $D_1, D_2, ..., D_K$ .In other words, if we use eqn. (6), then we have two assumptions:

1- Symptoms are independent among each other.
2- Diseases are mutually exclusive.

If the symptoms independence cannot be assumed, then conditional probability will be given by the following eqn.

$$P((S_1, S_2, ...S_j)|D_i) = P(S_1|D_i)P(S_2|D_i, S_1)P(S_3|D_i, S_1, S_2)....P(S_n|D_i, S_1, S_2, ...S_{n-1}).$$

Then we complete Bayes' formula for the complex dependent symptoms $S_1, S_2, ..., S_j$ and mutually exclusive diseases $D_1, D_2, ..., D_K$:

$$P(D_i / S_1, S_2, ...S_j) = \frac{P(D_i)P(S_1|D_i)P(S_2|D_i, S_1)P(S_3|D_i, S_1, S_2)....P(S_n|D_i, S_1, S_2, ...S_{n-1})}{\sum_{i=1}^{k} P(D_i)P(S_1|D_i)P(S_2|D_i, S_1)P(S_3|D_i, S_1, S_2)....P(S_n|D_i, S_1, S_2, ...S_{n-1})}. \quad (7)$$

In other words, if we use eqn. (7), we just have one assumption that diseases are mutually exclusive.

5 Design Structure of the Holonic Medical Diagnostic System under Uncertainty (HMDSuU)

In fact, the process of finding the best medical diagnosis from slight information from the user is a great challenge, whereas, Medical Diagnosis Decision Support HMAS under Uncertainty is one of the first systems that capable to reach this purpose. A large number of simple Agents, Swam Intelligent, Holonic paradigm, Bayes' theory, and Decision theory are elements required in specific functions to perform the diagnostic process. Possession of the diagnosis starts from the mediator agent, which is in the highest level of the hierarchy. Mediator agent is the importing point to the system that is capable to accept or reject the request according to its knowledge about the whole system and class of request. Fig. 3 illustrates the architecture of the holonic multi agent system based decision in a three level where mediator agent is the first one. Level two represents Disease Specialist Agents (DSA) that, in turn, plays the role as internal nodes of the hierarchy. The leaf level In turn, is Disease Representative Agents (DRA). They represent decision makers, which are specialists on a particular domain of class diseases.

DRA is capable to achieve the optimal diagnosis decision in a minimum total risk. During the diagnosis process multiple agents will emerge together to build Holon.

Multi simple agents communicated to pass through the blackboard technique. Two kinds of agent state in the middle and the leaf of the hierarchy, which, in turn, work together to find the optimal medical diagnosis decision through Holonic pattern.

In other words, HMDSuU is a system where a holon is a node in a holarchy and, at the same time, has a high degree of self-sufficiency. Indirect communication is the technique among agents for the purpose of coordination by using Stigmergy.

HMDSuU supports a medical institution in the procedure of decision optimal diagnosis and provides it with accurate information on the proportion of risk in case of a decision on the diagnosis.

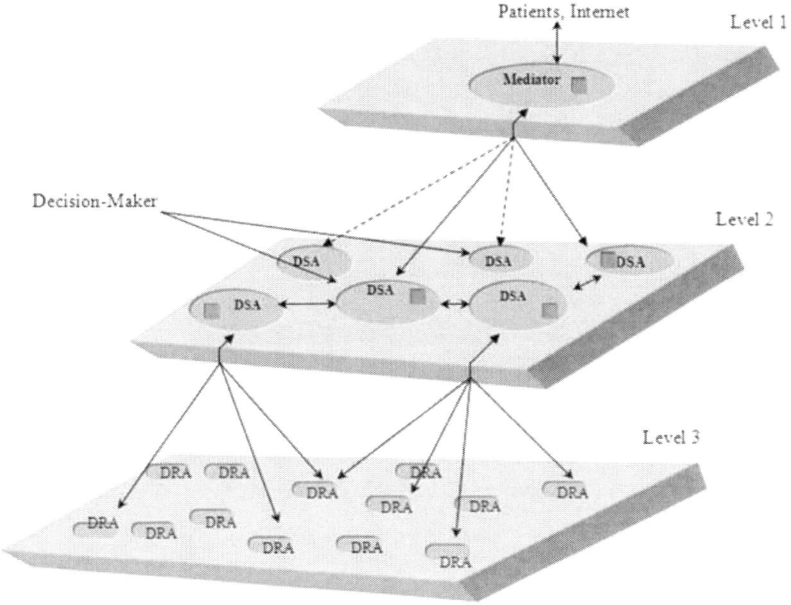

Fig. 3. Holonic Medical Diagnosis System

Whereby:
Random search - - - ->
Established route ⟶
DSA Diagnosis Specialist Agent
DRA Disease Representative Agent
▒ Blackboard

Furthermore, decision-making is an important part of all science, where specialists apply their knowledge in a given area to making decisions. Medical decision-making often involves making a diagnosis and selecting an appropriate treatment.

5.1 Diagnosis Finding (Decision-Making)

Pyramid of sequential decisions processes where a decision in each level is the decision in different situations. Base of the pyramid represents the decision under uncertainty because it is depends on the prior probability. In fact, probability in multi agent system represents the degree of agents' beliefs since an agent's decisions are based on its beliefs.

Gradually, away from, the base will get a higher accuracy of decision and in the same time percentage of lower risk until the optimal decision where the top of the pyramid represents is the last point of decision that represents the bayes risk (total risk). Middle steps are the levels of decision under risk, see Fig.4.

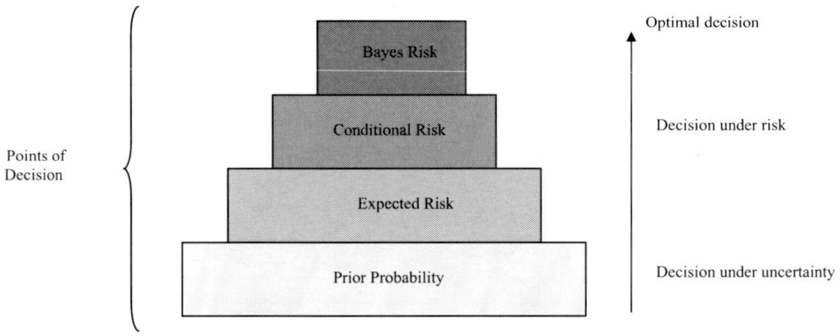

Fig. 4. Pyramid of Sequential Decisions

5.2 Diagnosis Finding

Decision making in HMDSuU depends on the strategies of bottom-up where the optimal decision starts from the leaf of the hierarchy. Fig.5 illustrates retrieved optimal decision starting from local to global optimal decision. Leaf agent returns the request (local optimal decision) on the form of diagnostic decision added to total risk. Highest level will receive the diagnostic decision with its total risk from multiple branches; afterward, it selects the local optimal decision that has minimum total risk. Finally, the global optimal decision will be selected from the agent mediator that received from a huge number of agents and from different disciplines.

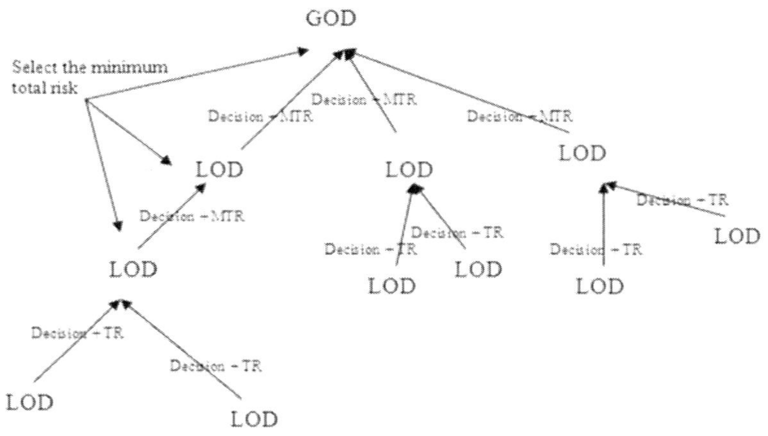

Fig. 5. Retrieve optimal decision

Where:

GOD Global Optimal Decision

LOD Local Optimal Decision

Note: The leaf agent takes its decision according to the Decision's Pyramid steps, but the higher level takes its decision according to selecting the minimum total risk that is sent from the previous level.

5.3 Activity Diagram of HMDSuU

Activity diagram of HMDSuU is demonstrated in Fig. 6, which is the cooperation procedure for medical diagnosis decision under uncertainty. Process starts from the request that is send from the user (medical institution) to the HMDSuU. Mediator agent received the request then decides whether accept the request or reject it depending on the capability of the system. In the case of accepting the request as an initial stage, mediator puts the request on its blackboard for finding diagnosis decision from the lower level. Each non-leaf agent has its own blackboard. The blackboard is like the pheromone trial in the ant that is one of the fundamental requirements for self-organization. Several DSAs can find the diagnosis or forward it to deeper knowledge agents. After that, if all symptoms are covered then DSAs will retrieve the diagnosis decision with zero total risk. If not, DSAs will declare the request on its blackboard to seek help from specialist agent that has an extra deep knowledge in an additional specialized area of diseases (DRAs).

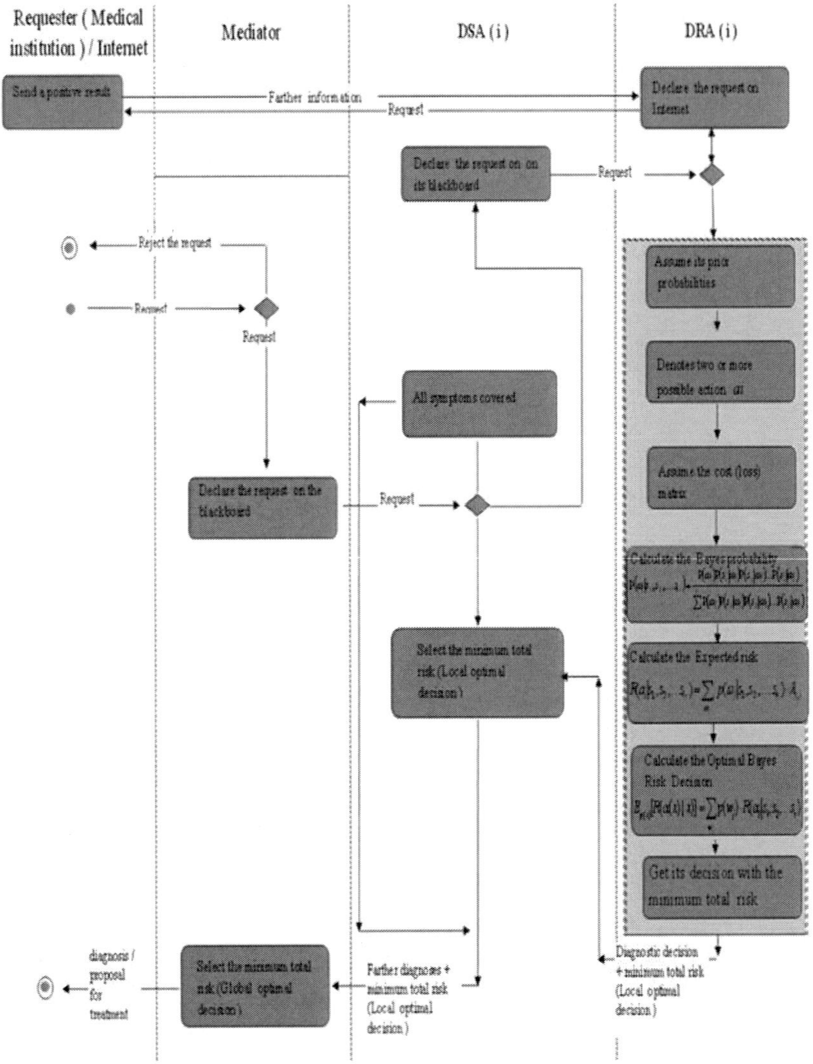

Fig. 6. Activity Diagram Of HMDSuU

DRAs are decision makers that find the optimal diagnosis decision in a minimum total risk by using bayes theory and decision theory.

In other side, DRAs use internet for obtaining additional information if it so requested. DRAs forward the local optimal diagnosis additionally with minimum total risk to high-level DSA. In this case, DSA selects local optimal diagnosis decision that is got from different DRAs, which have the minimum total risk.

Finally, mediator selects global optimal decision by filtering the retrieved request that comes from lower level and forward it to the medical institution.

Example

For the purpose of application integration between bayes theory and decision theory for finding the optimal medical diagnosis, we assume that we have five symptoms ($S_4, S_9, S_{15}, S_{28}, S_{77}$) as an input to the system. After filtering process of diseases inside DRA obtained three possible cases.

Table 1. Illustrates the final filtering of diseases according to the input symptoms

$P(S_i \vert D_j)$	D_{42}	$P(S_i \vert D_j)$	D_{55}	$P(S_i \vert D_j)$	D_{93}
#	S	#	S	#	S
0.4	S_4	0.025	S_4	0.12	S_4
0.01	S_9	0.07	S_9	0.33	S_9
0.009	S_{15}	0.5	S_{15}	0.09	S_{15}
0.3	S_{28}	0.096	S_{28}	0.18	S_{28}
0.1	S_{77}	0.17	S_{77}	0.046	S_{77}
#	S	#	S	#	S
#	S	#	S	#	S
1		1		1	

Where each agent has database, which in turn distinguishes it from other and embodied by:

1. Name of diseases (D)
2. Name of symptoms (S)
3. $P(S_i|D_j)$ Conditional probability of symptoms given diseases, which represents important the presentation of the disease
4. $P(D_i)$ Incidence (prevalence) of disease

Where table1 exemplifies filtering of diseases, and shaded cells are common symptoms after the trimming process.

Then DRA generates Cost (Loss) Matrix:

Cost (Loss) Matrix

	States of Nature				
Decision		w1	w2	w3	
	D_{42}	0	0.1667	0.1667	0.3333333
	D_{55}	0.1667	0	0.1667	0.3333333
	D_{98}	0.1667	0.1667	0	0.3333333
		0.33333	0.33333	0.333333	1

Prior probabilities were as follows:

$P(W_{1.}) = 0.264$

$P(W_2) = 0.0911$

$P(W_3) = 0.0974$

Calculate Bayes probability

$$\mathrm{P}(\omega_i | s_1, s_2, \ldots, s_r) = \frac{\mathrm{P}(\omega_i)\mathrm{P}(s_1|\omega_i)\mathrm{P}(s_2|\omega_i)\ldots\mathrm{P}(s_r|\omega_i)}{\sum_j^k \mathrm{P}(\omega_i)\mathrm{P}(s_1|\omega_i)\mathrm{P}(s_2|\omega_i)\ldots\mathrm{P}(s_r|\omega_r)}.$$

	P(Wj)*P(S4/Wj)*P(S9/Wj)*P(S15/Wj)*P(S28/Wj)*P(S77/Wj)
W1	2.8512E-07
W2	1.30091E-06
W3	2.87427E-06
SUM	4.46029E-06

P(Wj|S4,S9,S15,S28,S77)
0.063924034
0.291664168
0.644411798

Calculate expected risk

$$R(a_i \mid s_1, s_2, \ldots, s_r) = \sum_{\omega_j} p(\omega_j \mid s_1, s_2, \ldots, s_r) \cdot \lambda_{i,j} .$$

$R(a_i \mid S_4, S_9, S_{15} .S_{28} .S_{77})$
0.156012661
0.118055972
0.0592647

Calculate optimal decision

$$E_{p(x)}[R(\alpha(x) \mid x)] = \sum_{w_j} p(w_j) \cdot R(\alpha_i \mid s_1, s_2, \ldots s_r) \quad .$$

$R(a_i \mid S_4, S_9, S_{15} .S_{28} .S_{77})$ *P(Wj)
0.041187342
0.010754899
0.005772382

A decision function is optimal if it minimizes the total risk. Means that D_{98} is the optimal diagnosis. All the previous steps are the task for DAR agent and at the same time for local optimal diagnosis where the global optimal diagnosis decision takes just from the mediator of the HMDSuU.

6 Conclusion

The object of this study is to present a holonic medical diagnosis system, which unifies the advantages of decision theory under uncertainty with the efficiency, reliability, extensibility, and flexibility of the holonic multi agent system holonic paradigm.

Besides, HMDSuU is a system where a Holon is a node in a Holarchy with high self-organization. Indirect communication is the technique of coordination among agents by using Stigmergy. Moreover, HMDSuU in this paper is the challenge to solve the problem of uncertainty.

Uncertainty is a central feature in medicine generally and diagnosis particularly.

This paper investigates the feasibility of employing the aspects of holonic, multi agent system and swarm intelligence combined with the Bayesian theory and decision theory in order to reach the optimal medical diagnosis in fastest and shortest way with minimum cost.

References

[Aikens 83] Aikens, J.: PUFF: An expert system for interpretation of pulmonary function data. Computers and Biomedical Research 16, 199–208 (1983)

[Arus 06] Arus, C., Celda, B., Dasmahapatra, S., Dupplaw, D., Gonzalez-Velez, H., van Huffel, S., Lewis, P., Lluch-Ariet, M., Mier, M., Peet, A., Robles, M.: On the Design of a Web-Based decision Support System for Brain Tumour Diagnosis using Distributed Agents. In: 2006 IEEE/WIC/ACM International Conference on Web Intelligence & Intelligent Agent Technology (WI-IAT), Hong Kong (December 2006)

[Banu 08] Diri, B., Albayrak, S.: Visualization, and analysis of classifiers performance in multi-class medical data. Expert Systems with Applications 34, 628–634 (2008)

[Barnett 87] Barnett, G.O., Cimino, J.J., Hupp, J.A., Hoffer, E.P.: DXplain. An evolving diagnostic decision-support system. JAMA 258(1), 67–74 (1987)

[Barnett 96] Barnett, G.O., Hoffer, E.P., Packer, M.S.: DXplain-demonstration and discussion of a diagnostic decision support system. In: Proc. Annu. Symp. Comput. Appl. Med. Care, p. 822 (1996)

[Bravata 04] Bravata, D.M., Sundaram, V., McDonald, K.M., Smith, W.M., Szeto, H., Schleinitz, M.D., Owens, D.K.: Evaluating detection and diagnostic decision support systems for bioterrorism response. Emerging Infectious Diseases 10(1), 100–108 (2004)

[Catley 03] Catley, C., Frize, M.: A Prototype XML-Based Implementation of an Integrated 'Intelligent' Neonatal Intensive Care Unit. In: 4th IEEE Conference on Information Technology Applications in Biomedicine, UK (2003)

[Catley 03a] Catley, C., Frize, M., Walker, C.R., St. Germain, L.: Integrating Clinical Alerts into an XML-Based Health Care Framework for the Neonatal Intensive Care Unit. In: 25th IEEE EMBS, Cancun, Mexico (2003)

[Catley 04] Catley, C., Frize, M., Petriu, D.C.: Software Performance Engineering of a Web Service-Based Clinical Decision Support Infrastructure. ACM SIGSOFT Software Engineering Notes 29(1), 130–138 (2004)

[Catley 04a] Catley, C., Frize, M., Petriu, D.C., Walker, C.R., Yang, L.: Towards a Web Services Infrastructure for Perinatal, Obstetrical, and Neonatal Clinical Decision Support, Engineering in Medicine and Biology Society. In: IEMBS 26th Annual International Conference of the IEEE (2004)

[Charles 04] Charles, T.: Risk and Financial Management: Mathematical and Computational Methods, pp. 22–30. John Wiley & Son, Chichester (2004)

[Conrad 76] Conrad, P.: I identifying Hyperactive Children, pp. 51–66. Ashgate Publishing, Ltd (2006)

[DIL91] Dilts, D.M., Boyd, N.P., Whorms, H.H.: The Evolution of Control Architectures for Automated Manufacturing Systems. Journal of Manufacturing Systems 10(1), 79–93 (1991)

[Elhanan 96] Elhanan, G., Socratous, S.A., Cimino, J.J.: Integrating DXplain into a clinica information system using the World Wide Web. In: Proc. AMIA Annu. Fall, pp. 348–352 (1996)

[Feldman 91] Feldman, M.J., Barnett, G.O.: An approach to evaluating the accuracy of DXplain. Comput. Methods Programs Biomed. 35(4), 261–266 (1991)

[Frederick 05] Hillier, F.S., Lieberman, G.J.: Introduction to Operations Research, 8th edn., pp. 686–690. McGraw-Hill, Boston (2005)

[Foster 05] Foster, D., McGregor, C., El-Masri, S.: A Survey of Agent-Based Intelligent Decision Support Systems to Support Clinical Management and Research. In: Multi agent Systems for Medicine, Computational Biology, and Bioinformatics (July 2005)

[Hudson 02] Hudson, D.L., Cohen, M.E.: Use of intelligent agents in the diagnosis of cardiac disorders. Computers in Cardiology, 633–636 (2002)
[Iantovics 06] Iantovics, B.: A Novel Diagnosis System Specialized in Difficult Medical Diagnosis Problems Solving. In: Aziz- Alaoui, M.A., Bertelle, C. (eds.) Understanding Complex Systems, Emergent Properties in Natural and Artificial Dynamical Systems, pp. 185–195. Springer, Heidelberg (2006)
[Iantovics 07] Iantovics, B.: The CMDS Medical Diagnosis System, Symbolic and Numeric Algorithms for Scientific Computing, pp. 246–253. IEEE Computer Society Press, Washington (2007)
[James 85] James, B.: Statistical Decision Theory and Bayesian Analysis, pp. 10–32. Springer, Heidelberg (1985)
[Jerzy 91] Grzymala-Busse, J.W.: Managing Uncertainty in Expert Systems. Kluwer Academic Publishers, Dordrecht (1991)
[Kappen 02] Kappen, H.J., Neijt, J.P.: Promedas, a Probabilistic Decision Support System for Medical Diagnosis. Technical report, SNN - UMCU (2002)
[Klüver 03] Klüver, J., Stoica, C., Unland, R.: Multi agent Systems and Soft Computing Technologies: A promising symbiosis for reliable medical diagnosis. In: Proceedings of the International Joint Workshop on Soft Computing for Internet and Bioinformatics Frontiers, BISC FLINT-CIBI (2003)
[Koestler 67] Koestler, A.: The Ghost in the Machine. Hutchinson & Co., London (1967)
[Koestler 07] Sebastian, R., Nicolas, G., Vincent, H., Stéphane, G., Abderrafiâa, K.: An analysis and design concept for self-organization in holonic multi agent systems. In: Brueckner, S.A., Hassas, S., Jelasity, M., Yamins, D. (eds.) ESOA 2006. LNCS (LNAI), vol. 4335, pp. 15–27. Springer, Heidelberg (2007)
[Kulikowski 82] Kulikowski, C.A., Weiss, S.M.: Representation Of Expert Knowledge For Consultation: The CASNET And EXPERT Projects. In: Szolovits, P. (ed.) Arificial Intelligence In Medicine, pp. 21–55. Westview Press, Boulder (1982)
[Lemaire 99] Lemaire, J.B., Schaefer, J.P., Martin, L.A., Faris, P., Ainslie, M.D., Hull, R.D.: Effectiveness of the Quick Medical Reference as a diagnostic tool. CMAJ 161(6), 725–728 (1999)
[Lu 05] Lu, L.: Design and Implementation of Cooperative Distributed Dental Medical Information System. In: The 9th International Conference on Computer Supported Cooperative Work in Design Proceedings (2005)
[Lu 06] Lu, L.: A cooperative telemedicine environment for stomatological medical diagnosis. In: Proceeding s of the 2006 IEEE International Conference on Mechatronics and Automation, Luoyang, China, pp. 1647–1652 (2006)
[Lu 05a] Lu, L.: System design and development for a CSCW based remote oral medical diagnosis system. In: International Conference on Machine Learning and Cybernetics, August 18-21, vol. 6, pp. 3698 - 3703 (2005)
[Mabry 91] Mabry, M., Miller, R.: Distinguishing drug toxicity syndromes from medical diseases: a QMR computer-based approach. Computer methods and programs in biomedicine 35(4), 301–310 (1991)
[Matsumoto 04] Matsumoto, I., Shimada, Y., Kawaji, S.: Clinical diagnosis support system based on symptoms and remarks by neural networks. IEEE Cybernetics and Intelligent Systems 2, 1304–1307 (2004)
[Milho 00] Milho, I., Fred, A.L.N.: A user-friendly development tool for medical diagnosis based on Bayesian networks. In: Proceedings of the second International Conference on Enterprise Information Systems, Stafford, UK, pp. 176–180 (2000)

[Moreno 03] Moreno, A., Nealon, J.L.: Applications of Software Agent Technology in the Health Care Domain. Whitestein Series in Software Agent Technologies. Birkhäuser Verlag, Basel (2003)

[Shortliffe 76] Shortliffe, E.H.: Computer-Based Medical Consultations: MYCIN. Elsevier, New York (1976)

[Shieh 08] Shieh, J.S., Yang, Q.: Traditional Chinese medical diagnosis based on fuzzy and certainty reasoning. In: IT in International Symposium, pp. 295–300 (2008)

[Stensmo 96] Stensmo, M., Sejnowski, T.J.: Automated Medical Diagnosis based on Decision Theory and Learning from Cases. In: World Congress on Neural Networks, pp. 1227–1231 (1996)

[Timothy 04] Timothy, R.: Fuzzy Logic with Engineering Applications, pp. 326–330. John Wiley and Sons, Chichester (2004)

[Ulieru 00] Ulieru, M., Cuzzani, O., Rubin, S.H., Ceruti, M.G.: Application of Soft Computing Methods to the Diagnosis and Prediction of Glaucoma. In: Proc. of the 2000 IEEE International Conference on System, Man, and Cybernetics, SMC 2000, Cybernetics Evolving to Systems, Humans, Organizations, and their Complex Interactions, Nashville, TN, USA, October 8-11 (2000)

[Ulieru 02] Ulieru, M., Geras, A.: Emergent Holarchies for e-Health Applications: A Case in Glaucoma Diagnosis. In: Proc. IECON 2002, HOL - Agent-based Intelligent Automation and Holonic Control Systems, Sevilla (November 2002)

[Ulieru 03] Ulieru, M.: Internet-Enabled Soft Computing Holarchies for e-Health Applications. In: Zadeh, L.A., Nikravesh, M. (eds.) New Directions in Enhancing the Power of the Internet, pp. 131–166. Springer, Berlin (2003)

[Ulieru 03a] Ulieru, M.: Internet-Enabled Soft Computing Holarchies for e-Health Applications. In: Zadeh, L.A., Nikravesh, M. (eds.) Fuzzy Logic and the Internet. Physica Verlag, Heidelberg (2003)

[Ulieru 03b] Ulieru, M., Cuzzani, O., Rubin, S., Ceruti, M.: Application of Soft Computing Methods to the Diagnosis and Prediction of Glaucoma. In: 2000 IEEE International Conference on Systems, Man and Cybernetics, SMC 2000, Cybernetics Evolving to Systems, Humans, Organizations, and their Complex Interactions, Nashville, TN, USA, October 8-11, pp. 3641–3646 (2000)

[Ulieru 06] Ulieru, M., Unland, R.: A Stigmergic Approach to Medical Diagnosis. In: AAMAS, Japan (2006)

[Unland 03] Unland, R.: A Holonic Multi agent System for Robust, Flexible, and Reliable Medical Diagnosis. In: Meersman, R., Tari, Z. (eds.) OTM Workshops (2003)

[Unland 05] Unland, R., Ulieru, M.: Swarm Intelligence and the Holonic Paradigm: A Promising Symbiosis for Medical Diagnostic Systems Design. In: Khosla, R., Howlett, R.J., Jain, L.C. (eds.) KES 2005. LNCS (LNAI), vol. 3682, pp. 154–160. Springer, Heidelberg (2005)

[Unland 05b] Unland, R., Stoica, C., Klüver, J.: A Holonic Medical Diagnosis System Based on MAS Technology and Neural Networks. Journal Special Issue on Computational Intelligence for Bioinformatics (2005)

[wikipedia] `http://en.wikipedia.org/wiki/Medical_diagnosis`

[Yang 04] Yang, L., Frize, M., Eng, P., Walker, R.C., Catley, C.: Towards Ethica Decision Support and Knowledge Management in Neonatal Intensive Care in 26th IEEE EMBS (2004)

[Yang 08] Yang, Q., Shieh, J.S.: A multi agent prototype system for medical diagnosis. In: 3rd International Conference on Intelligent System and Knowledge Engineering, ISKE, vol. 1, pp. 1265–1270 (2008) (ail orders only)

Curriculum Vitae

Israa Al-Qaysi is research assistant at the Institute for Computer Science and Business Information Systems, Section Data Management Systems and Knowledge Representation, of the University of Duisburg-Essen. She received her M. Sc. in Statistics at the University of Baghdad. She worked six years as lecturer in Baghdad Universities. Her research experiences include Decision theory, Accelerated failure-Time, Survival Fractions, and Multi Agent System.

Rainer Unland is a full professor in computer science at the Institute for Computer Science and Business Information Systems (ICB) at University of Duisburg-Essen where he heads the chair *Data Management Systems and Knowledge Representation*. He has authored, co-authored and edited numerous publications, journals and (text)books in the areas of non-standard/object-oriented database management systems, XML and database systems, object-oriented software development, component-based and aspect-oriented software engineering, advanced transaction management, computer supported cooperative work, (distributed) artificial intelligence, especially Multi agent Systems, and industrials informatics. Moreover, he has served as Chair and/or PC member for more than 100 national and international conferences, workshops, and symposia. He is co-founder of the annual International German Conference on Multi agent Systems Technology (MATES) and the annual International conference SABRE that serves as an umbrella conference for topics related to software engineering, multi agent system, Grid computing, and Web-Services and the Internet. Moreover, he is servers on several editorial boards of other computer science related journals.

Claus Weihs holds the chair for Computational Statistics at the department of statistics of the Dortmund University of Technology, Germany. He worked for more than nine years as a statistician in chemical industry (CIBA-Geigy, Switzerland). He received his Ph.D. in Mathematics from the Department of Mathematics of the University of Trier, Germany. His research interests include classification methods, engineering statistics, statistical process control, statistical design of experiments, time series analysis, and statistics in music data analysis.

Cherif Branki Professor Branki has an enviable record of research and development in the provision of innovation and technological support and advice to numerous organisations including global/international concerns and also Scottish SMEs.

In particular, Professor Branki has developed a track record in research and development as well as recent and current management of several international projects:COSMOS- Construction On Site Mobile Operation Support (a 4.5 Million Euros ESPRIT European Funded project), PATRICIA-Performance and Theory of Remote Intelligent Cooperative Agents on the Internet (DAAD: German-British Council supported project), MAST- Multi agent s in Structural Design (A Polish-British Council Project). He has worked as senior investigator in several national and international projects such FOCUS (Front-end for Open and Closed User Systems), the first UK multimedia project: MUMS (Multi Media User Modelling Systems) and CEMS (Customisable Extranet Management System) as a KTP.He has provided technological support and advice to numerous SMEs including Tier Technologies Ltd (UK) a proof of concept using a wireless interface to a corporate database to support the business traveller, as well as agent based workflow system for CEMAG GmbH (Germany) Ltd.

Part II

Rehabilitation Decision Support Systems

Chapter 6
A Data Mining Approach for Predicting the Pregnancy Rate in Human Assisted Reproduction

Loris Nanni[1], Alessandra Lumini[1], and Claudio Manna[2]

[1] Department of Electronic, Informatics and Systems (DEIS),
Università di Bologna,
Via Venezia 52, 47023 Cesena, Italy
Tel.: +39 0547 339121
{loris.nanni,alessandra.lumini}@unibo.it
[2] Genesis Center for Reproductive Medicine, Via Velletri 7, 00198 Roma, Italy
manna@genesisclinic.org

Abstract. One of the most relevant aspects in human assisted reproduction is to decide if, at a given moment, the endometrium is receptive for embryo implantation, in order to perform embryo transfer cycle or to postpone it in another cycle. This might increase both patients' convenience and the cost-effectiveness of the assisted reproduction procedure. To help human experts in taking this decision, we developed an artificial intelligence system based on a data mining approach where data extracted from the endometrium/subendomentrium and their vascularization are evaluated. The proposed system has been tested on a dataset of 62 cycles of intracytoplasmic sperm injection (ICSI) and several machine learning methods are compared for obtaining a high performing system. Particularly interesting is the performance obtained considering only three features: the patient's age, the subendometrial volume and the endometrial vascularization/flow index; the best system, based on a random subspace of decision tree, obtains an area under the ROC curve (AUC) of 0.85 in predicting the pregnancy rate. These preliminary results show that it is possible to measure in a non invasive way a set of features from a patient, for assisting the decision of making or postponing the embryo transfer.

1 Introduction

Nowadays there is a growing interest by physicians and biologists in studying an important social problem such as the human infertility and intensive research is being done in the field of human assisted reproduction (HAR) for performing in vitro fertilization (IVF)/intracytoplasmic injection (ICSI).

The most important contributing factors to achieve a successful pregnancy by IVF are the quality and number of oocytes/embryos, uterine receptivity, and age of the woman. In contrast to the high success rate in oocyte retrieval and fertilization, embryo implantation is the most frustrating step, failing in most patients transfer. Moreover, in

S. Brahnam & L.C. Jain (Eds.): Adv. Comput. Intell. Paradigms in Healthcare 5, SCI 326, pp. 97–111.
springerlink.com

spite of the progress made in the recent years concerning controlled ovarian stimulation, oocyte retrieval and fertilization, the techniques of uterine embryo transfer and the criteria to assist the decision of making or retarding it remain quite unchanged and the implantation rate per embryo is still very low [23].

Several attempts have been made to support human assisted reproduction by means of machine learning techniques based on image analysis or data mining. In particular, promising results have been obtained for oocytes/embryos selection by some works based on a non-invasive examination of the oocytes/embryos [20][9][15][16]. One of the major problems in designing oocytes/embryos selection techniques is to collect a large and reliable dataset to training the classifiers: unfortunately, the classes of the collected images can be assigned with certainty only if all the n transferred embryos/oocytes gave rise to no births or to n births.

Another possibility is to analyze the images of the endometrium and other clinical data of the patient to develop a data mining approach for giving a pregnancy outcome in patients undergoing IVF. An attractive property of this problem, with respect to the previous one, is that it is easy to create a reliable training set for training an artificial intelligence technique, since the extracted features (endometrium/clinical data) are directly related with each cycle of a patient. Therefore they can be labeled with certainty as belonging to one of the existing classes (cycle ending with pregnancy/cycle with a negative outcome).

Section 2 reviews some results about the evaluation of different factors (e.g. endometrial thickness, endometrial pattern, hormonal profile and other data) for predicting pregnancy outcomes in patients undergoing IVF. A fair comparison among all published results is very difficult due to the different acquisition conditions, dimensions of the study, reported conclusions. In particular at this time there is no agreement on conclusions: for example about the significance of the endometrium thickness in predicting the pregnancy.

In conclusion, since it is very difficult to evaluate the at this time there is no agreement on the significance of a single different factors in predicting the pregnancy,; in this work we are interested in developing an automated system that can support this decision using more factors together, without the constraints of invasive (and expensive) analyzes.

The aim of this study is to evaluate measures related to an IVF-ICSI cycle (i.e. age of the patient, endometrial and subendometrial vascularization indexes, etc.) to verify if they are good predictors to distinguish patients who became pregnant from the others who were not successful.. To this aim we do not limit our analysis to the statistical significance but we propose a data mining approach trained starting from such features, obtained by evaluating and comparing different machine learning approaches. Our best system is based on a random subspace of decision trees and obtains a very interesting area under the ROC curve of 0.85 in predicting the pregnancy rate.

2 Literature Review

The success of an in vitro fertilization/embryo transfer (IVF/ET) treatment is strictly related to several factors including the choice of good quality embryos, successful ovarian stimulation, the method of assisted fertilization and the culture conditions. In particular the evaluation of the receptivity of the endometrium can be useful in assist the decision of making or retarding the embryo transfer. Different strategies have been developed to evaluate endometrial receptivity, Some invasive, such as the histologic dating of an endometrial biopsy, endometrial cytokines in uterine flushing, the genomic study of a timed endometrial biopsy, and some are non-invasive, such as the ultrasound examination of the endometrium which evaluates several factors including endometrial thickness, endometrial pattern, endometrial volume, endometrial blood flow.

Many results have been reported [17] about the evaluation of different factors (e.g. endometrial thickness, endometrial pattern, hormonal profile and other data) [10] for predicting pregnancy outcomes in patients undergoing IVF. Unfortunately, there is no agreement on conclusions: for example, some studies have shown that the pregnancy rate increases once the endometrium thickness attains a particular threshold [7], while others have yielded contrasting findings [22]. In fact, it is not easy to define a reliable criterion to decide if in a particular moment a uterus is well-suited to receive an embryo.

Several studies have shown that some ultrasound parameters of the endometrium and the presence of a blood supply towards the endometrium can be useful predictors of the uterine receptivity for embryo transfer after in vitro fertilization [14]. Nevertheless, controversial results have been published about the possibility of using such measures as IVF outcome predictors [3].

For example the authors of [13] found that 3D power Doppler endometrial vascularization indexes are statistically significant in predicting the pregnancy rate, while other investigators [5][18] did not reached the same conclusions.

Several recent works have investigated measures of the endometrial and subendometrial regions and their statistical significance to the implantation rating: in [12] the absence of color Doppler mapping at the endometrial and subendometrial levels has been associated to a significant decrease in the implantation rate, whereas in [26] the presence of vessels reaching the subendometrial halo and the endometrium has been related to an increased pregnancy rate, in [8] a comparison of different measures is carried out showing that the subendometrial flow index (obtained by 3D power Doppler ultrasonography) and subendometrial vascularization flow index on the day of human chorionic gonadotropin administration are better than the endometrial volume in predicting pregnancies in IVF cycles.

The presence of conflicting results with regard to the role endometrial and subendometrial blood flows in the prediction of pregnancy in IVF treatment can be explained by several reasons, mainly related to the differences in the dataset creation protocols. In particular there is no consensus on the acquisition procedure, on the day when the ultrasound examination for assessing endometrial receptivity should be done and on the rules for the selection of the subendometrial region.

Most of the published works are related to small datasets (ranging from 35 to 90) and are related to patients with different characteristics (e.g. in [25] are examined patients aged <38 years), and different day of ultrasound examination (probably more related to logistic reasons than to the physiological changes of endometrial blood flow throughout the menstrual cycle). For example, the following days of ultrasound examination are reported: the day of hCG [27], oocyte retrieval [5][18] and blastocyst embryo transfer [8]. Another difference among studies is the definition of subendometrial region that can be considered [17] to be within 1, 5 or 10 mm of the endometrial contour.

Researchers are still uncertain whether the main reason of the contradictory findings reported in many studies is the difference in the collection of the datasets, anyway in order to make comparable the future studies it should be appreciable the definition a common testing protocol.

To this aim, further studies are needed to determine the change in endometrial and subendometrial blood flows from late follicular phase to early luteal phase in order to select the best day of ultrasound examination: a possible result could be that a series of measures could be more significant than a single measure to delineate the role of endometrial and subendometrial blood flows in predicting IVF outcome. Finally, to the best of our knowledge, all the published works analyzes all the factors considered singularly, without taken into account their possible interaction. In this work we approach this problem by a machine learning technique, thus considering the best combination of features able to predicting IVF outcome.

3 Materials and Methods

3.1 Study Design

The experiments have been carried out on a dataset containing some clinical data from M=62 cycles of ICSI, each related to a different patient, resulting in 27 successes (pregnancy) and 35 failures (non-pregnancy). The clinical data collected for each cycle are described in table 1; the information related to vascularization and the measures of the endometrium have been collected the the day of hCG administration. In figure 1 we report some samples of endometrial images from which the features F7-F10 are extracted.

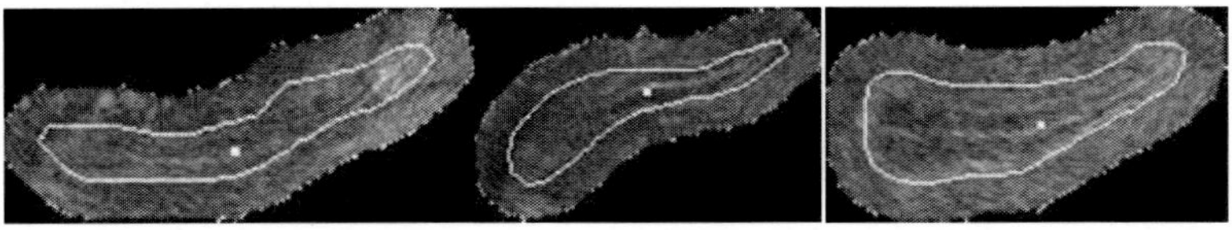

Fig. 1. Some samples of endometrial images (with also the sub-endometrium)

Table 1. Clinical data extracted from each patient

Index	Name	Description	Range
F1	Age	Age of the woman	24 - 45
F2	Endometrial vascularization index	Presence of blood vessels (vascularity) in the endometrium	0- 8.96
F3	Endometrial flow index	The mean power Doppler signal intensity inside the endometrium, to express the average intensity of flow	0- 31.16
F4	Endometrial vascularization/flow index	It is a combination of vascularity and flow intensity inside the endometrium	0- 3.03
F5	Sub-endometrial vascularization index	It measures the presence of blood vessels (vascularity) in the subendometrium	0 - 6.42
F6	Sub-endometrial flow index	The mean power Doppler signal intensity inside the subendometrium, to express the average intensity of flow	0 - 41.76
F7	Sub-endometrial vascularization/flow index	It is a combination of vascularity and flow intensity inside the subendometrium	0 - 3.82
F8	Endometrial thickness	The thickness of the endometrial region	6 - 14.2
F9	Endometrial volume	The volume of the endometrial region	1.46-9.09
F10	Sub-endometrial volume	The volume of the sub-endometrial region	2.52-17.76

3.2 System Proposed

The proposed system is based on a data mining approach trained by clinical information related to the patient (age, vascularization and endometrial measures). We have tested several classification systems and a feature selection technique for selecting the most important features. The best results have been obtained by a random subspace of decision trees trained with 3 selected features. The architecture of the best system is schematized in figure 2, while a description of the each step is given in the following sub-sections.

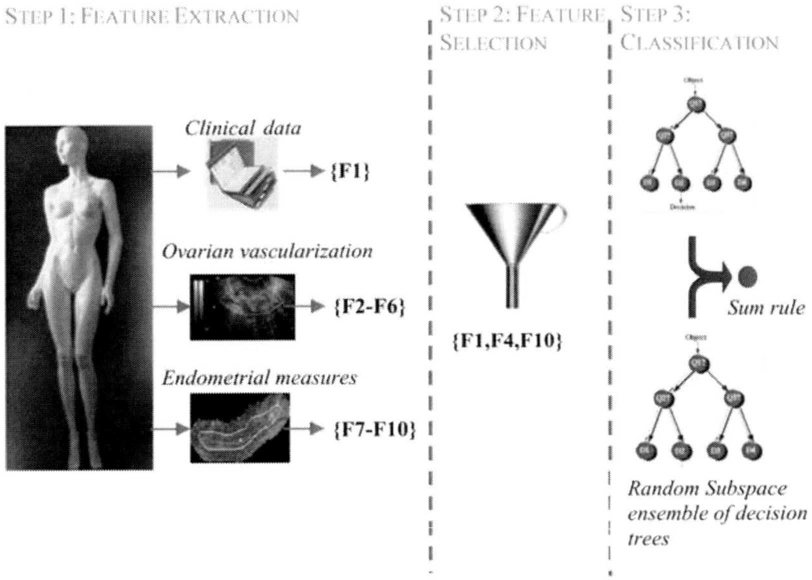

Fig. 2. Proposed system for predicting pregnancy outcomes in patients undergoing IVF

3.3 Feature Extraction

The set of features extracted for each cycle/patient are listed in table 1. All the ultrasound scans and measurements were performed on the day of hCG administration by the same observer with the digital platform VOLUSON i System (Zipf, Austria) provided with a volumetric multifrequency vaginal probe (3 to 9 MHz) that has an insonation angle of 146°. The power Doppler sample was placed over the endometrial longitudinal section, including the whole endometrial and subendometrial areas, maintaining the same characteristics in all examinations: normal quality of color, color gain -3.4, wall motion filter of 50 Hz and pulse repetition frequency of 300 Hz. The acquisition of the uterine volume is performed by placing the volume box, with a scanning angle of 90°, just over the previous power Doppler image, ensuring that a complete uterine volume had encompassed the entire endometrium and subendometrium.

The maximum endometrial thickness was obtained from the longitudinal or ''A'' plane and was defined as the greatest distance between both myoendometrial interfaces. The built-in VOCAL Imaging Program for the 3D power Doppler histogram analysis was used to calculate the endometrial volume (VOL) and thickness (TH) and indices of blood flow within the endometrium. Vascularization index (VI) has been obtained measuring the ratio of the number of color voxels to the number of all the voxels; it represents the presence of blood vessels (vascularity) in the endometrium and is expressed as a percentage of the endometrial volume.

Flow index (FI), the mean power Doppler signal intensity inside the endometrium, expresses the average intensity of flow. Vascularization/flow index (VFI) is a derived measure calculated by multiplying VI and FI [19]. During the analysis and calculation, the manual mode of the VOCAL Contour Editor was used to cover the whole 3D volume of the endometrium with a 15° rotation step. Hence, 12 contour planes were analyzed for the endometrium of each patient to cover 180°. Following assessment of the endometrium itself, the subendometrium was examined through the application of 'shell-imaging', which allows the user to generate a variable contour that parallels the originally defined surface contour. In the present study, the subendometrial region was considered to be within 5 mm of the originally defined myometrial–endometrial contour. VI, FI and VFI of the subendometrial region were obtained accordingly.

3.4 Feature Selection

A feature selection step is performed in order to choose the most proper feature for this problem. The selection is performed according to the well-known sequential forward floating selection (SFFS)[1] method, that is based on the optimization of a fitness function (in this case the performance of the classification system in terms of AUC). On the basis of the experimental results reported in figure 5, the number of features to be maintained has been fixed to d=3.

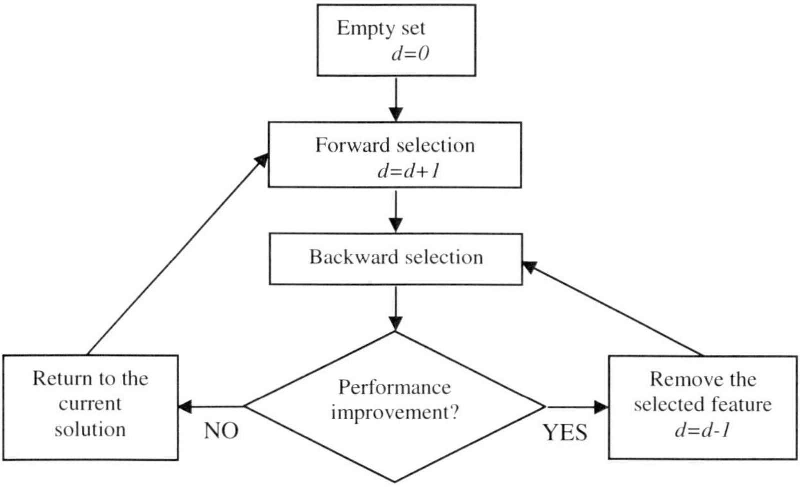

Fig. 3. Flowchart of the SFFS procedure

[1] Implemented as in PRTools 3.1.7 Matlab Toolbox.

SFFS is a bottom up search procedure introduced by Pudil et al. [21] consisting of a forward search-step and a conditional backward search-step. The forward search-step starts from an initially empty set of features and successively adds features from a set of original candidates in order to optimize the fitness function. Each time a single feature is added, a backward search-step is performed that identifies the least significant feature in the current feature set and removes it unless it is the last feature added. In figure 3 a flowchart of SFFS is reported.

3.5 Classification

Several general purpose classifiers have been proposed in the literature [1], in this work we use decision trees (figure 4), since, due to their instability, they are particularly suited to be combined in an ensemble. A decision tree (DT) is a decision support tool in the form of a tree structure [1]. The goal of the tree is to create a model that predicts the value of a target label based on several input features. Each interior node (decision node) corresponds to one of the input features and specifies a test to be carried out on a single feature, the edges to children represent all the possible outcome of the test of that input feature and indicate the path to be followed, each leaf node indicates the value of the target label given the values of the input features represented by the path from the root to the leaf. A tree can be "trained" by splitting the source set into subsets based on a test on a single feature. This process is repeated on each derived subset in a recursive manner called recursive partitioning. The recursion is completed when the subset of the training patterns at a given node all has the same label, or when splitting no longer adds value to the predictions.

In this work we have used a decision tree with pruning[2], where the information gain is used as binary splitting criterion.

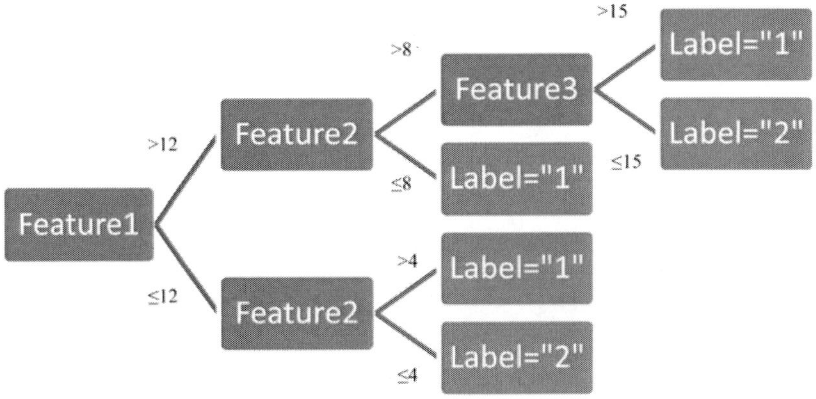

Fig. 4. Representation of a decision tree

[2] Implemented as in PrTools 3.1.7
`ftp://ftp.ph.tn.tudelft.nl/pub/bob/prtools/prtools3.1.7`

To improve the performance of the system an ensemble method is designed based of the combination of decision trees. The literature is full of studies showing that ensembles enhance the performance of many stand-alone classifiers [6], in particular if they are composed of highly accurate and diversified classifiers. Among the several methods proposed to obtain diversity among each classifier of the ensemble, one of the most used is the random subspace method (RSM) [4], which is based on the idea of training each classifier using a different feature set. Random subspace is a technique that modifies the training set reducing its dimensionality (in terms of features) by randomly sampling subsets of the features. The accuracy of the ensemble is thus enhanced by aggregating the resulting base classifiers, each trained on a modified training set. RSM assembles classifiers by applying the following three steps:

1. Given a d-dimensional labeled dataset $D = \{\mathbf{x}_i, y_i\}$, $\mathbf{x}_i \in \Re^d$, $y_i \in C$, n new projected k-dimensional training sets $D_j=\{P_j(\mathbf{x}_i), y_i\}$ are generated, where $P_j : \Re^d \rightarrow \Re^k$ is a random projection, obtained by random selecting k of the d features.
2. Each new training set D_j is given in input to a fixed classifier H_j;
3. The final ensemble H is obtained by aggregating the base classifiers $H_1 \ldots H_n$ through a given decision rule (the sum rule, in this work).

In this work we use RSM for creating an ensemble of n=50 classifier, each trained on a subspace of dimension k=2 of the original feature space (d=3, after feature selection).

4 Experimental Results

As a preliminary result in table 2 the mean, standard deviation and statistical correlation (p-value) of the 10 features according to the well-known Fisher exact test [2] are reported. Fisher's exact test is a statistical test used to determine if there are nonrandom associations between two categorical variables. A statistically significant association between the two variables is observed if their P-value is lower than 0.05.

It is clear that the best feature is F5, the subendometrial VI; this result is also confirmed by the test with the area under the ROC curve, reported in table 4. Another interesting result is that the endometrial thickness is not useful to discriminate between the two classes, according to the findings in [22] but in contrast to [7].

In this section the result of several experiments aimed at validating the proposed approach on the available dataset are reported. The experiments are performed according to the leave-one-out testing protocol [1], which involves the use of a single observation from the original samples as testing data, and the remaining observations as training. This is repeated M times, such that each of the M observations in the dataset is used once as testing data.

Table 2. Comparison of features between pregnant/non-pregnant groups

Index	Name	Pregnant (Mean ± Sdt)	Non-Pregnant (Mean ± Sdt)	P-value
F1	Age	35.37 ± 3.88	37.48 ± 5.46	0.11
F2	Endometrial VI	1.30 ± 1.95	0.31 ± 0.45	0.12
F3	Endometrial FI	21.59 ± 9.68	19.49 ± 9.60	0.12
F4	Endometrial VFI	0.44 ± 0.74	0.08 ± 0.12	0.12
F5	Sub-endometrial VI	2.59 ± 1.90	1.28 ± 1.16	**0.03**
F6	Sub-endometrial FI	29.73 ± 5.07	27.65 ± 6.23	0.30
F7	Sub-endometrial VFI	1.04 ± 0.97	0.48 ± 0.45	0.30
F8	Endometrial TH	9.71 ± 1.71	9.74 ± 1.89	1.00
F9	Endometrial VOL	3.86 ± 1.58	3.96 ± 1.44	0.21
F10	Sub-endometrial VOL	11.03 ± 2.65	10.59 ± 2.64	0.60

As performance indicator we use the area under the ROC curve (AUC) [24]. The AUC is a scalar measure of performance which can be interpreted as the probability that the classifier will assign a lower score to a randomly picked positive sample (i.e. a cycle resulting in pregnancy) than to a randomly picked negative sample (i.e. a failed cycle).

The first test is aimed at comparing different data mining approaches for the analysis of the clinical data. Several methods are compared in table 3:

- **SVM**: a linear Support Vector Machine classifier [1] trained by data linearly normalized to [0,1];
- **NN**: a stand-alone nearest-neighbor classifier [1] with the original features linearly normalized to [0,1];
- **DT**: a stand-alone decision tree trained by the original features (not linearly normalized);
- **RSSVM**: a random subspace ensemble of n=50 Support Vector Machines, each trained on a subspace of dimension k=6 of the original linearly-normalized feature space (d=10, without feature selection);
- **RSNN**: an ensemble method based on a random subspace of n=50 nearest neighbor classifiers, each trained on a subspace of dimension k=6 of the original linearly-normalized feature space;
- **RSDT**: an ensemble method based on a random subspace of n=50 decision trees, each trained on a subspace of dimension k=6 of the original non-normalized feature space;
- **ROTB**: a RotationBoosting of n=50 decision trees; the RotationBoosting is a recently proposed method for the creation of ensembles that has been proven [27] to outperform other state-of-the-art ensembles in several classification problems.

Table 3. Data mining results

Method	AUC
SVM	0.69
NN	0.55
DT	0.62
RSSVM	0.64
RSNN	0.64
RSDT	0.69
RotB	0.64

The best performance, obtained by RSDT and SVM, is quite interesting: an AUC of 0.69 in a small dataset means that the set of features is useful for solving this difficult problem.

The second test is aimed at evaluating the significance of the different features by considering the features one-by-one and by applying a feature selection approach (i.e. the SFFS described in section 2.5). The rationale of this experiment is to show that the order of selection of a feature can be influenced by the correlation among features and can be different by the "discriminant power" of the feature itself [21]. For that reason we can expect better performance considering features in groups than evaluating them singularly. The evaluation of the "discriminant power" of each feature is performed by measuring the AUC obtained by each single feature (table 4, column 3). The three best features selected by SFFS for the RSDT approach are highlighted in table 4, column 4; notice that some good features are not selected, since SFFS chooses a set of three features considering an objective function (the maximization of AUC), while the "discriminant power" simply reports the AUC of each feature without considering its correlation with the others.

Table 4. Evaluation of the significance of the features

Index	Name	Discriminant Power	Selected
F1	Age	0.6344	Yes
F2	Endometrial VI	0.6847	No
F3	Endometrial FI	0.6243	No
F4	Endometrial VFI	0.6772	Yes
F5	Sub-endometrial VI	0.7032	No
F6	Sub-endometrial FI	0.6132	No
F7	Sub-endometrial VFI	0.6698	No
F8	Endometrial TH	0.5132	No
F9	Endometrial VOL	0.5492	No
F10	Sub-endometrial VOL	0.5000	Yes

Finally, the third experiment is aimed at choosing the optimal value *d* of selected features by SFFS; in figure 5 a comparison among the performance of two approaches (SVM and RSDT) is reported as a function of *d*. It is clear that the best method is the random subspace of decision trees for *d*=3 (where each subspace contains 2 features).

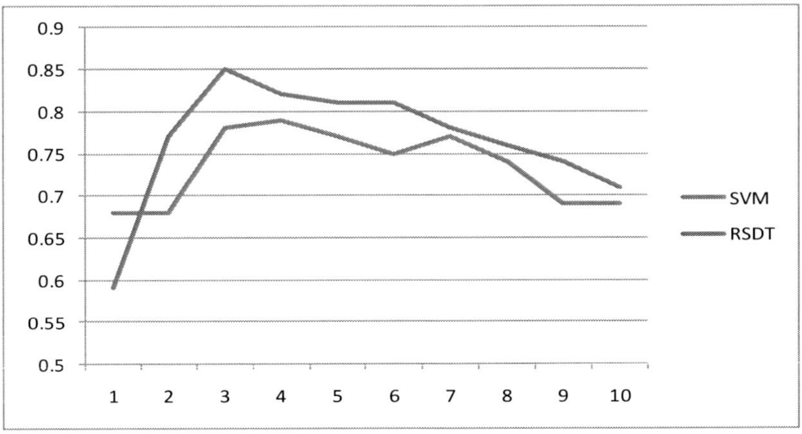

Fig. 5. AUC of SVM and RSDT as a function of *d* (features selected by SFFS)

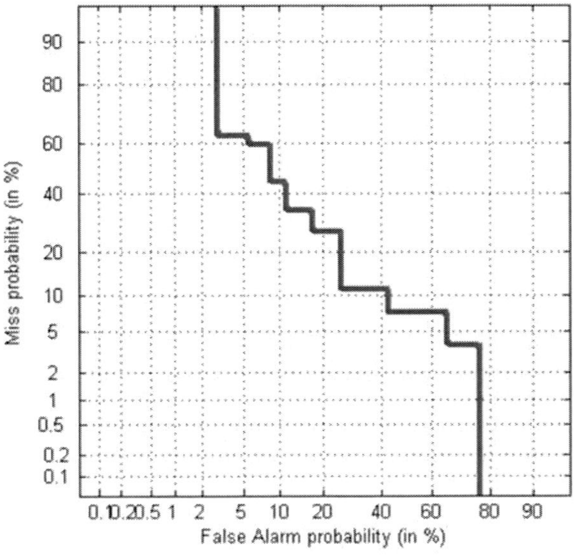

Fig. 6. DET-curve obtained by the proposed system

In order to confirm the benefit of our method the DET curve of RSDT has also been considered. The DET curve [11] is a two-dimensional measure of classification performance that plots the percentage of false alarm (i.e. false positive) against the miss probability (i.e. false negative). An interesting finding from this curve is that fixing an operative threshold such as the miss probability is around the 10%, a false alarm probability is detected, that is discarding one over 10 possibly good cycles the probability of failures is less than 30%.

5 Discussion

This paper focused on the study of non-invasive techniques to decide if an endometrium demonstrates maximal receptivity for embryo implantation. To take this decision, we developed a system based on the age of the patient, on information extracted from endometrium and from follicles vascularization. The results of our analysis can be useful to decide if trying to fecundate a patient in a given moment, or in case of a negative prognostic factor, suggesting to freeze eggs for their possible use in more receptive endometrial situations.

The supporting decision system proposed in this work has been tested considering the leave-one-out testing protocol using a dataset of 62 cycles of intracytoplasmic sperm injection (ICSI) related to 62 women. Our results are very encouraging considering that we have obtained an area under the ROC curve of 0.85, which means that in 85% of the cases our system is able to assign a higher score to a receptive endometrium with respect to a non-receptive one.

Our main practical finding is that it is possible to obtain a reliable enough method, based on a set of features measured in a non invasive way from a patient, that can help physicians and biologists in assisting the decision of making or retarding the embryo transfer. The most similar work on this subject is that of Mercè et al. [13]. These authors reached with AUC curve a predictive value of 0.82 for endometrial Flow Index but only when no grade I embryo or only one were transferred. Our results were irrespective of number and grade of transferred embryos. The inclusion of these parameters could improve the performance, though without them the uterine factor is better isolated and its importance in the reproductive outcome becomes more understandable. However patient's age is mostly related to oocyte and consequently to embryo quality. Our experiments confirm other results published in the literature which are based on the analysis of stand-alone features: *(i)* two widely used factors like the endometrium thickness and volume, measured in the day of hCG administration, are not useful in this decision problem [22]; *(ii)* the vascularization data measured from both the endometrium and the subendometrium in the day of hCG administration, are significant for this prediction problem [25].

As future work we plan to test the proposed method on a larger dataset, and using clinical data extracted in different periods. Moreover, since the failure of an ICSI cycle is related to different factors, such as endometrial receptivity and oocyte/embryo quality, we plan, as future work, to train our supporting decision system also considering the information extracted from the embryos and oocytes.

References

1. Duda, R., Hart, P., Stork, D.: Pattern Classification. Wiley, New York (2001)
2. Fisher, R.A.: On the interpretation of $\chi 2$ from contingency tables, and the calculation of P. Journal of the Royal Statistical Society 85(1), 87–94 (1922)
3. Friedler, S., Schenker, J.G., Herman, A., Lewin, A.: The role of ultrasonography in the evaluation of endometrial receptivity following assisted reproduction treatments: a critical review. Hum Reprod Update 2, 323–335 (1996)
4. Ho, T.K.: The random subspace method for constructing decision forests. IEEE Transactions on Pattern Analysis and Machine Intelligence 20(8), 832–844 (1998)
5. Jarvela, I.Y., Sladkevicius, P., Nelly, S., Ojha, K., Campbell, S., Nargung, G.: Evaluation of endometrial receptivity during in-vitro fertilization using three-dimensional power Doppler ultrasound. Ultrasound Obstet. Gynecol. 26, 765–769 (2005)
6. Kittler, J., Hatef, M., Duin, R.P.W., Matas, J.: On Combining Classifiers. IEEE Transactions on Pattern Analysis and Machine Intelligence 20(3), 226–239 (1998)
7. Kovacs, P., Matyas, S., Boda, K., Kaali, S.G.: The effect of endometrial thickness on IVF/ICSI outcome. Hum. Reprod. 18, 2337–2341 (2003)
8. Kupesic, S., Bekavac, I., Bjelos, D., Kurjak, A.: Assessment of endometrial receptivity by transvaginal color Doppler and three-dimensional power Doppler ultrasonography in patients undergoing in vitro fertilization procedures. J. Ultrasound Med. 20, 125–134 (2001)
9. Manna, C., Patrizi, G., Rahman, A., Sallam, H.: Experimental results on the recognition of embryos in human assisted reproduction. Reprod. BioMed. Online 8, 460–469 (2004)
10. IJland, M.M., Hoogland, H.J., Dunselman, G.A.J., Lo, C.R., Evers, J.L.H.: Endometrial wave direction switch and the outcome of in vitro fertilization. Fertility and Sterility 71(3), 476–481 (1999)
11. Martin, A., et al.: The DET curve in assessment of decision task performance. In: Proc. of EuroSpeech, pp. 1895–1898 (1997)
12. Maugey-Laulom, B., Commenges-Ducos, M., Jullien, V., Papaxanthos- Roche, A., Scotet, V., Commenges, D.: Endometrial vascularity and ongoing pregnancy after IVF. Eur. J. Obstet. Gynecol. Reprod. Biol. 104, 137–143 (2002)
13. Mercè, L.T., Barco, M.J., Bau, S., Troyano, J.: Are endometrial parameters by three-dimensional ultrasound and power Doppler angiography related to in vitro fertilization/embryo transfer outcome? Fertility and Sterility 89(1) (2008)
14. Mercè, L.T.: Ultrasound markers of implantation. Ultrasound Rev. Obstet. Gynecol. 2, 110–123 (2002)
15. Morales, D.A., Bengoetxea, E., Larrañaga, P.: Selection of human embryos for transfer by Bayesian classifiers. Comput. Biol. Med. 38, 1177–1186 (2008)
16. Morales, D.A., Bengoetxea, E., Larrañaga, P., García, M., Franco, Y., Fresnada, M., Merino, M.: Bayesian classification for the selection of in vitro human embryos using morphological and clinical data. Comput. Methods Prog. Biomed. 90(2), 104–116 (2008)
17. Ng, H.Y.Y., Chan, C.C.W., Tang, O.S., Yeung, W.S.B., Ho, P.C.: The role of endometrial blood flow measured by three-dimensional power Doppler ultrasound in the prediction of pregnancy during in vitro fertilization treatment. European Journal of Obstetrics & Gynecology and Reproductive Biology 135(1), 8–16 (2007)

18. Ng, E.H.Y., Chan, C.C.W., Tang, O.S., Yeung, W.S.B., Ho, P.C.: The role of endometrial and subendometrial blood flows measured by three-dimensional power Doppler ultrasound in the prediction of pregnancy during IVF treatment. Hum. Reprod. 21, 164–170 (2006)
19. Pairleitner, H., Steiner, H., Hasenoehrl, G., Staudach, A.: Three- dimensional power Doppler sonography: imaging and quantifying blood flow and vascolarization. Ultrasound Obstet. Gynecol. 14(2), 139–143 (1999)
20. Patrizi, G., Manna, C., Moscatelli, C., Nieddu, L.: Pattern recognition methods in human-assisted reproduction. Int. Trans. Oper. Res. 11, 365–379 (2004)
21. Pudil, P., Novovicova, J., Kittler, J.: Floating search methods in feature selection. Pattern Recognition Letters 15(11), 1119–1125 (1994)
22. Puerto, B., Creus, M., Carmona, F., Civico, S., Vanrell, J.A., Balasch, J.: Ultrasonography as a predictor of embryo implantation after in vitro fertilization: a controlled study. Fertil. Steril. 79, 1015–1022 (2003)
23. Rashidi, B.H., Sadeghi, M., Jafarabadi, M., Tehrani Nejad, E.S.: Relationships between pregnancy rates following in vitro fertilization or intracytoplasmic sperm injection and endometrial thickness and pattern. Eur. J. Obstet Gynecol. Reprod. Biol. 120, 179–184 (2005)
24. Fawcett, T.: ROC Graphs: Notes and Practical Considerations for Researchers. HP Laboratories, Palo Alto (2004)
25. Wu, H.M., Chiang, C.H., Huang, H.Y., Chao, A.S., Wang, H.S., Soong, Y.K.: Detection of the subendometrial vascularization flow index by threedimensional ultrasound may be useful for predicting the pregnancy rate for patients undergoing in vitro fertilization-embryo transfer. Fertil. Steril. 79, 507–511 (2003)
26. Zaidi, J., Campbell, S., Pittrof, R., Tan, S.L.: Endometrial thickness, morphology, vascular penetration and velocimetry in predicting implantation in an in vitro fertilization program. Ultrasound Obstet. Gynecol. 6, 191–198 (1995)
27. Zhang, C.-X., Zhang, J.-S.: RotBoost: a technique for combining Rotation Forest and AdaBoost. Pattern Recognition Letters (2008), doi: 10.1016/j.patrec.2008.03.006

Chapter 7
Agent-Based Monitoring of Functional Rehabilitation Using Video Games

Stuart T. Smith[1], Amir Talaei-Khoei[2], Mililani Ray[3], and Pradeep Ray[2]

[1] Neuroscience Research Australia
s.smith@neura.edu.au
[2] Asia-Pacific ubiquitous Healthcare Research Centre (APuHC),
School of Information Systems, Management and Technology,
Australian School of Business
University of New South Wales (UNSW), Australia
amirtk@student.unsw.edu.au, p.ray@unsw.edu.au
[3] University of Western Sydney, Australia

Abstract. In recent years, there has been an increasing trend towards using video games for health applications. In particular interactive video games, where an individual interacts with the game by moving their limbs or whole body, have started to find application in the field of rehabilitation medicine. The often dull and repetitive nature of rehabilitation exercise can be transformed into an activity to which patients happily adhere via the use of engaging video games that are enjoyable to play. One additional potential benefit of video game use in rehabilitation is that patients can continue to interact with the video game system in their own home following discharge from hospital. As such, video games may offer a means for rehabilitation specialists to remotely assess compliance of patients with their rehabilitation therapy and monitor changes in function over time. Although the use of technology for monitoring health at home is now widespread, an as yet unexplored challenge lies in integrating information technologies with rehabilitation games. This keeps the health professional informed about compliance and progress of the video game exercise, while the patient performs her/his prescribed rehabilitation routine at home. Therefore, there is a strong need for a computational framework to support the medical professional and patient by using an agent-based architecture. Agents are pieces of software that act on behalf of human roles, involved in rehabilitation process. The objective of this chapter is to thus address major issues in designing an agent-based mobile monitoring system for rehabilitation treatments. The chapter also suggests how to remotely measure the patient's progress in rehabilitation treatments while the patient plays video games at home.

Keywords: Functional Rehabilitation, Video Game, Mobile Health Monitoring, Software Agent.

S. Brahnam & L.C. Jain (Eds.): Adv. Comput. Intell. Paradigms in Healthcare 5, SCI 326, pp. 113–141.
springerlink.com

1 Introduction

In the past two decades there has been a significant transformation in our understanding of the extent to which functional recovery is possible following damage to central and peripheral nervous systems. In parallel with advances in the neuroscience of nervous system recovery, the engineering professions have witnessed recent developments in wireless sensing, virtual reality and computer gaming technologies. A quick search using the terms "video game" and "rehabilitation" in any internet search engine will reveal a number of media reports of the use of games platforms such as the Nintendo Wii in aged-care or rehabilitation settings. While video games are clearly being used to engage patients in activities outside of normal rehabilitation practice, in the scientific literature, there are relatively fewer published reports on the effect of video game play on improving performance in functionally impaired individuals. The current lack of objective data concerning the effectiveness of video games in rehabilitation may in part reflect the fact that many off-the-shelf games are simply too difficult for patient groups to effectively use in attaining rehabilitation goals. Furthermore most, if not all, commercially available video games provide little more than a rudimentary method (eg highest scores) for tracking progression of performance changes over time.

Before video games can become truly effective in facilitating rehabilitation, it is suggested that the games need to be developed with both the functional limitations of patients "players" as well as the goals of rehabilitation medicine in mind. For this to happen, as much as possible, the intelligence of rehabilitation practitioners, such as physical and occupational therapists, needs to be built into agents within the game. These agents will also need to provide physical (or cognitive) challenge to the patient, tracking of performance changes over time and motivation to continue with rehabilitation tasks, especially when rehabilitation is done in the home away from the guidance of specialists. This chapter aims explore how design and development of video games in a rehabilitation, rather than purely entertainment, context might occur. It is important that game developers and information technology specialists are made aware of the requirements of the health sector and that rehabilitation specialists are similarly aware of the possibilities offered by technological (video game) solutions. As such the aim of Section 2 of this chapter is provide technologists with an introduction to the process of rehabilitation of brain and nervous system injury. To build a bridge between information technologists and health researchers, Section 3 presents an overview of the ways in which recent advances in virtual reality and video gaming technology have already been leveraged by health researchers and practitioners. Section 4 aims to inform rehabilitation specialists in particular, and health practitioners more generally, about the possibilities offered by mobile computing and information technology and how development of home-based rehabilitation games might best be developed. Finally, Section 5 presents a usability evaluation framework for mobile health monitoring of home-based rehabilitation games while Section 6 discusses implications of the research, postulates about new directions for research in the area and concludes the chapter.

2 Rehabilitation of Brain and Nervous Systems

2.1 Stroke and Spinal Cord Injury

Damage to the brain and central nervous system by stroke or injury is frequently associated with significant functional impairment for the individual. Stroke is one of the leading causes of death and disability throughout the world [59], and is the leading cause of disease burden in countries such as Australia [66] and the United States. A recent survey of community-dwelling adults in the United States [11] found that 44% of patients who had suffered a stroke reported having limitations in most, if not all, activities of daily living (such as bathing, cooking, dressing), most of which require the coordinated efforts of posture, head and limb control strategies. Significant impairments in the activities of daily living are also prevalent in individuals with spinal cord injury (SCI). Recent figures show that there are between 721 and 906 cases of SCI per million of population in the USA, corresponding to between 183,000 and 230,000 persons [51].The physical and functional impact of spinal cord injury will vary according to both the type and level of the injury. The type of SCI is generally classified into two categories, complete and incomplete injuries. A complete injury occurs with a total severance of the spinal cord, and there is a total loss of motor and sensory function below the level of injury. Complete spinal injuries are always bilateral, i.e.: affecting both sides of the body equally, and voluntary movement and physical sensation are absent below the level of injury. An incomplete spinal cord injury occurs with a partial severance of the spinal cord, and the individual will still retain some sensation below the level of the injury. The functional effects of an incomplete injury are variable, and the individual may have more function on one side of the body than the other [99].

2.2 Rehabilitation of Stroke and SCI

The rehabilitation of stroke and spinal cord injury patients can be best understood in terms of being an ongoing collaborative process between the individual and their care givers, which aims to restore them to their maximum potential in all areas of life [46]. In practice, rehabilitation interventions employ a dual strategy to achieve this aim. First, there is the restorative approach that aims to restore an individual's highest level of functional ability, according to their level of injury. And secondly, there is the compensatory approach that addresses ways of compensating for any shortcomings in function by using adaptive techniques, such as lowering the level of kitchen countertops to make wheelchair access easier, or by using equipment, such as electric wheelchairs [99]. Individuals in rehabilitation are encouraged to reach the highest level of expected functionality for their level of injury by accomplishing a series of functional goals. These goals are set in conjunction with the patient's care team and aim to teach individuals new ways to manage their daily activities, and can include such tasks as eating, dressing and eating.

Success in achieving these functional goals is affected not only by an individual's physical abilities, but also by their general health, coping skills and psychological well-being. To successfully manage the various influences on therapeutic outcome, the rehabilitation of SCI in a hospital setting involves the collaboration of a number of professionals across a range of different rehabilitation services [10]. This multi-disciplinary healthcare team, in collaboration with the patient, will plan and structure a patient's goals, and regularly communicate about their' progress to ensure that treatment is effective. Typically, a patient's rehabilitation experience will involve care by medical and nursing staff, who are responsible for all aspects of a patient's ongoing health issues, physiotherapists, who will help optimise a patient's physical capacity and mobility, psychologists, who will assess a patient's cognitive and sensory abilities, and assist them in adjusting to their new circumstances, and occupational therapists, who train the patient to become as independent as possible in carrying out their activities of daily living. The efforts of this healthcare team are supported by community liaison services who will help ease the patient's transition back into the community after discharge from hospital.

2.3 The Role of the Occupational Therapist in Rehabilitation

Occupational therapy is focused on helping patients to reach the highest level of physical and psychological independence that their injuries, homes and work environments will allow [46]. This is achieved through the use of purposeful and meaningful activities, such as stirring dough to make cookies, or picking up and sorting small coins. These exercises are designed to both assist in a patient's physical rehabilitation, and also encourage and motivate them to participate fully during therapy. They also help to improve a patient's physical coordination and dexterity, as well as increase the range of motion, strength and endurance of their limbs. Purposeful and meaningful activities also improve a patient's problem solving strategies, so that they may be able to successfully deal with the everyday challenges their condition brings [99].

Occupational therapists work with a range of individuals, who, for whatever reason have difficulty in accessing or performing the activities they require to lead meaningful and satisfying lives. The role of the therapist in rehabilitation includes assessing a patient's functional ability and selecting a variety of tasks for the patient to practice in order to restore, or compensate, for loss of function in a particular area. The therapist may also act as coach during the process of rehabilitation, demonstrating how to complete a given task, and also providing feedback on a patient's performance [37]. Each patient will engage in an individualized program during their rehabilitation, which is designed to improve their ability to perform everyday activities, and can include retraining to eat, dress, wash, cook and even drive an adapted vehicle. Occupational therapists also provide for a vocational assessment, to prepare the client for re-entry back into the community, and review their options for returning to work. To further support a patient's move back into the community a liaison OT will also visit a patient's potential home and job site and recommend how these can be adapted for optimal use.

2.4 Engaging Patients in Rehabilitation Therapy

In occupational therapy, rehabilitation of function this is achieved through the use of purposeful and meaningful activities such as completing a jigsaw to train fine hand movements, or throwing and catching a ball to promote motor coordination. It is the meaningful and purposeful nature of these activities that are the key therapeutic qualities of an occupational therapy intervention, as it is purposefulness that organises behaviour, while meaningfulness that motivates performance [98]. Given that a patient's daily program of rehabilitation will typically involve three or more hours of physical and occupational therapy, motivation is an important component in therapy, enabling them to engage at their maximum capacity, and derive the greatest benefit from their' rehabilitation.

A patient's level of motivation is widely accepted as a key indicator of the success of inpatient rehabilitation interventions [60], yet there exists an inherent difficulty in defining and measuring such an abstract component of human performance. Lenze and colleagues [57] suggest a more useful alternative is to measure the level of participation in therapy, as participation is an overt behaviour which can be directly observed and quantified. Examining a patient's participation level in rehabilitation has the added benefit of allowing clinicians to document not just the quantity, but more importantly, the quality of a therapeutic intervention. A further study by Lenze and colleagues [56] suggests that the level of a patient's functional outcome in physical therapy is directly related to their participation during[56] rehabilitation. These researchers observed 242 hospital inpatients, with a variety of physical impairments, during their rehabilitation, and found that those who were rated with higher levels of participation in therapy showed a higher percentage of functional improvement (as indexed by the Functional Independence Measure; [48] and had a shorter length of stay in hospital than those who were rated as having lower levels of participation. Although this study did not examine participation levels for each patient category, and comparisons across impairments can be problematic, it does indicate that the level of participation has an impact of the functional benefits of regular and repeated therapy.

High levels of patient participation are also desirable during occupational therapy, especially when retraining a patient to perform activities of daily living (ADLs), such as grooming, eating, bathing and dressing. The more successful a patient is at acquiring the skills to perform these activities the greater opportunities they will have to function independently when returning to the community. Having the highest possible level of independence can also help the patient to foster a wide range of social and leisure activities, enabling them to live more satisfying and meaningful lives [5]. In practical terms too, the more independent a patient is the less their physical condition will be experienced as a handicap, and the more capable they will be in pursuing their own interests in terms of education, employment and family life.

According to Christiansen [13] the level of participation in occupational therapy can also contribute to a patient's psychological well-being, as occupational therapy presents them with an opportunity to choose activities that express their individual identities, allowing self-actualization and providing a platform for self-expression. This view is also supported by Rebeiro and Cook [81] who suggest that the experience of occupational engagement can result in a positive spin-off in terms of mental health and overall well-being. These findings have particular importance for the rehabilitation of SCI patients, considering the high incidence of depression among the patient population [53]. Depression can act as a confounding factor in therapy, and patients with depression have been found to require longer periods of rehabilitation [85]. Higher levels of participation in rehabilitation therefore appear to be a vital element in successful therapeutic outcomes, both in terms of improving a patient's overall health, but also in the development of functional abilities and practical life-skills.

2.5 The Problem of Motivation

Traditionally, the purposeful activities designed to encourage participation in OT have involved the use of handicrafts such as basket weaving, wood carving, and sewing. These activities, aimed at developing sensory and motor coordination, are, by their very nature repetitive and tend to be tedious if not varied over the course of a therapeutic program [99]. As a therapeutic medium these activities are functional, but present a limited appeal to a modern patient population, and it is more common today to find a computer or games console in a family home than traditional craft activities. In instances where the patient population is overwhelmingly young and male [73], these craft activities may also be particularly unsuitable to fully engage them in their rehabilitation. Society has changed dramatically since the early days of occupational therapy, and so too have the interests and expectations of patients who attend for rehabilitation. Yet these interests and expectations need to be considered if patients are to be encouraged to participate at an optimal level during their therapy.

Conventional occupational therapy interventions are also less than ideal from a clinical perspective, as they provide little opportunity for grading the level of task difficulty, and so may be too difficult for patients beginning rehabilitation, and yet fail to challenge more able patients [51]. These activities are also limited in their capacity to encourage the development of dynamic balance, which entails maintaining balance and equilibrium while in motion, a skill that is essential in carrying out activities of daily living, from shopping to driving a car. Given the limitations of conventional occupational therapy activities and the importance of keeping patients engaged and motivated in therapy, it is an ever present challenge for therapists to find activities that are meaningful to the patient, yet still possess a therapeutic value. In the following section we explore how video games are beginning to be used to address the issue of patient compliance and motivation, especially with regard to rehabilitation.

3 Video Games for Health

The following presents a brief overview of the relationship between video game use and various health outcomes. Evidence for and against the benefits of video game use is presented as well as suggestions for future developments that will lead to increased exploration of this technology in the health domain.

In the popular media, as well as the scientific research literature, the playing of video games has often been associated with negative health outcomes such as increased aggression and violence [2], problems with addiction to gameplay [31], social withdrawal [28], increased sedentary behaviour [35], increased risk of cardiovascular problems [32] and even increased risk of epileptic seizures [14]. With the popularity of active gaming systems such as the Nintendo Wii, there has also been a rise in reports of "Wii knee" [84], central palmer blisters [106], haemothorax [76] and ruptured tendons [8].

Despite the gloom surrounding the negative health consequences of engaging in video gameplay, there is an increasing interest in the potential application of video game and virtual reality technology to various health domains. A quick search using the terms "video", "games", "medicine, "rehabilitation", "pain" and "health" on the primary medical research database available from the US National Library of Medicine (http://www.pubmed.gov) reveals over 1000 research articles, many of which report significant beneficial effects of the application of video games to health. The following, far from exhaustive, list of examples provides a flavor of how widely video games are being used in health contexts:

3.1 Games for Health Education and Training

The use of video games in health is one example of the emerging use of games for "serious" applications. Serious games offer an alternative to traditional means of informing and educating people across a range of domains from medicine to the military [7]. In health contexts, video games have been used to: train surgeons in laparoscopic surgery [87], teach children about a range of health and dietary issues [58], educating medical students about fall risk in older people [23] through to improving cancer-related knowledge in adolescents with cancer [6].

3.2 Games for Healthy Weight

Many "exergame" or interactive gaming systems that are commercially available have had significant impact on the increasing problem of obesity and diabetes in children, adolescent and adults. Video games are being used to promote healthy diets in young adults [77], increase energy expenditure in young children [29], promote physical activity and decrease sedentary time [63] as well as promote weight loss among overweight children and adolscents[28] and increase overall fitness [103].

3.3 Games for Pain Distraction

One of the most interesting uses of video games is as a distraction therapy for the treatment of pain. Pain tolerance (in response to a cold pressor stimulus) has been shown to be improved while children and young adults [2] play video games. The fear of pain (needlestick) in children has also been shown to be significantly reduced while children play self-distracting video games [104]. Distracting video games have also been shown to significantly ameliorate the subjective level of pain experienced by children in pediatric burns units during dressing changes [38].

3.4 Virtual Reality as a Rehabilitation Tool

In recent years one of the emerging rehabilitation tools that appears to meet the challenge of finding therapeutic interventions that are both purposeful and motivating, is the use of virtual reality (VR) technology [44]. Virtual reality systems involve the use of a three dimensional computer simulation of the real world, or imaginary space, and allow the user to engage with this simulated environment through the use of various multimedia peripherals such as a keyboard and mouse, joystick controller, video camera tracking, inertial sensors (accelerometers), cybergloves and dance mat. Most recently, the Nintendo Wii controller has become a popular, low-cost method for providing individuals with an engaging virtual reality input device. Users experience virtual environments by interacting with displayed images, moving and manipulating virtual objects, and performing other actions in a way that engenders a feeling of actual presence and immerses their senses in the simulated environment. Users are provided with visual, audio and, in some instances, haptic (i.e.: tactile), feedback of their performance to further enhance the experience [69].

Although virtual reality applications have been used in research and entertainment applications since the 1980's, it was only during the late 1990's that VR systems began to be developed and studied as potential tools to enhance and encourage participation in rehabilitation [1]. And the use of virtual reality in rehabilitation has slowly been expanding since then, and is now being used successfully as a treatment and assessment tool in a wide variety of applications, most notably in the fields of motor, and cognitive, rehabilitation. For example, Merians and colleagues [67] found that exercise conducted using a virtual reality interface enhanced the training of hand movements in patients post stroke, resulting in improved function of the fingers, thumb, and overall range of motion. The researchers also found that these improvements were later transferred to real world tasks, demonstrating that VR based therapy has the potential to encourage a level of exercise intensity and participation that is comparable to conventional interventions.

Virtual reality has also been used successfully in the cognitive rehabilitation of patients with traumatic brain injury (TBI). Grealy and colleagues [30] for example, conducted research trials with TBI patients which required them to navigate around a variety of virtual environments, and found that patients performed better than no-exercise controls on verbal and visual learning tasks, as well as demonstrating improved reaction times. The researchers were able to conclude that exercising in a virtual environment offered the potential for cognitive gains; however it is not clear if the gains would have been observed using the same exercises in a conventional environment. It is also uncertain if the gains achieved were transferred outside the experimental setting, or lasted longer than the duration of the study. Virtual environments can also be used as a flexible assessment tool to safely determine patients' levels of ability in a variety of real world tasks prior to their return to a community setting, for example. Cristiansen and colleagues. [13] found that a virtual reality kitchen proved to be effective in assessing the ability of TBI patients to operate safely in such an environment during a meal preparation task. Even though the research involved a prototype virtual environment it does highlight the potential utility of virtual reality in the training of very practical skills and patterns of behavior that will allow patients to function successfully in the real world.

Although these examples provide only a brief overview of the variety of applications of virtual reality in rehabilitation, the end goal of these initiatives is to encourage and motivate patients to participate to their maximum capacity during therapy, and thereby develop the skills they need to function in their own real world environments in a more independent manner. Weiss and colleagues [51] suggest that virtual reality platforms provide a number of unique advantages over conventional therapy in trying to achieve this aim. First, virtual reality systems provide ecologically valid scenarios that elicit naturalistic movement and behaviors in a safe environment that can be shaped and graded in accordance to the needs and level of ability of the patient engaging in therapy. Secondly, the realism of the virtual environments allows patients the opportunity to explore independently, increasing their sense of autonomy and independence in directing their own therapeutic experience. Thirdly, the controllability of virtual environments allows for consistency in the way therapeutic protocols are delivered and performance recorded, enabling an accurate comparison of a patient' s performance over time. And lastly, virtual reality systems allow the introduction of "gaming" factors into any scenario to enhance motivation and increase user participation [39]. The use of gaming elements can also be used to take patients' attention away from any pain resulting from their injury or movement. This occurs the more a patient feels involved in an activity and again, allows a higher level of participation in the activity, as the patient is focused on achieving goals within the game [90].

3.5 VR Video Gaming Systems for Home Rehabilitation

While the use of VR technology has been proven to be effective in laboratory or clinical based settings, the equipment used is often expensive, requires expert users and has a dedicated purpose. Furthermore, once a patient returns to their home environment following acute rehabilitation care, partial and unmet rehabilitation needs may ultimately lead to a loss of functional autonomy, which increases utilization of health services, number of hospitalizations and early institutionalization, leading to a significant psychological and financial burden on the patients, their families and the health care system [101]. The potential for rehabilitation at home will enable patients can tailor their program of rehabilitation and follow individual schedules, potentially leading to a reduction in subsequent health care service provision. Undergoing treatment at home gives people the advantage of practicing skills and developing compensatory strategies in the context of their own living environment. By leveraging the connectivity enabled by broadband technology and video game technology, it should be possible to build distributed communities of individuals undergoing rehabilitation as well as providing a mechanism for remote measurement and assessment of function. The following section reviews how video game technology has started to be used in a health context and then goes on to discuss how mobile agent technology can add value to video game systems that can be utilized for home-based rehabilitation.

In the following sections we will outline how video game technologies could potentially be combined with mobile communication technologies to develop a "virtual" occupational therapist that can both engage patients in rehabilitation exercise once they have returned home from acute care as well as monitoring changes in functional ability over time.

4 Mobile Monitoring in Home-Based Rehabilitation

Governments and healthcare agencies today are focussing on information technology as a means to cut costs and improve quality of care. The current approach in e-health is mobile solutions that support patients in different kinds of treatments such as rehabilitation. This allows patients to stay at theirs homes or residential sets during their medical care period [91].

This section focuses on use of mobile technologies in health monitoring for supervised home-based rehabilitation treatments. Section 0presents an overview on mobile technologies. Section 0presents the potential use of mobile technologies in healthcare domain. This section also defines mobile health monitoring as a way to increase the role of OT while patients are participating in given treatments at their homes. Section 4.3 presents how methods in the field of computer supported cooperative work design mobile heath monitoring systems to enhance cooperation in home-based rehabilitation treatments.

4.1 Mobile Computing

Recent advances in mobile networks and the necessity of processing data during transit have led to anytime and anyplace service delivery. Tremendous growth of pervasiveness of technology and increasing trends towards small and portable devices, such as mobile phones, PDAs and the like, creates the demand for another approach to process information and deliver services, called *mobile computing*. The falling cost of mobile computing devices has allowed complex cooperation and communication patterns across geographical areas. As a consequence, mobile computing has made a paradigm shift in the way people use computing technologies in their everyday lives.

Mobile computing implies wireless transmission, but wireless transmission does not necessarily imply mobile computing. Wireless transmission mentions that the device should be able to react in a specific way in various situations instead of delegating this task to some general purpose distributed entities. The idea replaces the Remote Invocation (RI) to Remote Execution (RE). In Remote Invocation, the computing device sends required data to the server through massage passing to execute a certain process on the server. Therefore, each transaction requires at least two acts of communication: request and acknowledgment. Communication by data exchange in RI requires both parties to remain on-line during the transaction. The computing device and server should also get agreed on a protocol in advance. In order to overcome the difficulties of using RI, in remote execution, the computing device does not only call the process on the server but also provides the process for itself. In other words, each call contains the executable process and its arguments. In RE, both, the computing device and the server, should be agree on a language instead of a protocol.

4.2 Mobile Computing and Healthcare

Recent comprehensive market studies [41,27,64,62] show that mobile computing has recently been involved in health care setting. Gregg Malkary, Managing Director, Spyglass Consulting Group [62] states "Mobile computing in healthcare is poised to revolutionize the way medicine is practiced at the point of care. Mobile devices enable clinicians to access patient information quickly, efficiently and securely from any location and at any time." This market can be divided in three segments [62]: (1) Health record Solutions: This segment is defined by using mobile computing to access medical records and informational materials. (2) Enterprise systems integration: This segment includes integrated computing to access clinical and financial information anywhere and anytime. (3) Legacy systems integration: This segment is characterized by solving a specific task or business process, which requires integration with clinical systems. Legacy systems require:

- *Cooperation*: Healthcare processes involve various roles and agencies who must cooperate. These roles, called *cooperative roles* [9] - are typically distributed across geographical areas. Here, cooperation addresses the situation that roles individually and independently interact together to achieve a common goal [36]. The need for cooperation is highlighted when a process spans across multiple agencies [16]. In such a healthcare process, the integrated system must support a cooperative knowledge based environment that facilitates cooperation considering relevant information leading to the successful resolution of the process.
- *Communication*: According to what we mentioned above, cooperative roles need to exchange relevant information to facilitate cooperation. Therefore, along cooperation, they also need to communicate. Since roles are geographically dispersed, in order to avoid having sporadic contacts, mobile communication is beneficial. This technology supports cooperative roles and ensures that the process can be handled in the most effective and efficient way possible.

The market research [62] predicts that legacy segment is going to grow the fastest over the next coming years. The study states that departmental healthcare systems are already in place and store much of the clinical information. On the other hand, clinicians still need to be assisted in some medical processes such as tracking patients at their homes. The use of mobile computing, in order to track home-based treatments, is one of the contributions of *Mobile Health Monitoring*.

4.3 Mobile Health Monitoring

Schwaibold and et al. [91] believe that "To enhance the quality of treatment for those people [patients], it is vital to enhance the quality of their monitoring first, so those instructions for nutrition and treatment can be optimized and the patient might be informed faster." Today, one problem in healthcare is insufficient availability of patient information while she/he is out of physical access. In addition, the period of time that decisive vital signs can be measured is also long. This concern has led to the use of mobile computing in health monitoring systems, called Mobile Health Monitoring (MHM). These kinds of systems are increasingly seen as an effective method of providing patient care. MHM allows for continuous transmission of patient information such as vital sign or treatment progress to doctors. Furthermore, the management of chronic diseases has long been recognized as an application of mobile monitoring [61,83].

Magrabi and et al. [61] have developed a web-based system for home monitoring in cystic fibrosis. The system provides a standard browser which gets activated whenever new patient data is sent. The system, based on comparison and analysis with the patient's history, sends reminders and suggestions to the doctor and patient via email. In this system, the need of automation for data entry by body-attached sensors has been ignored. Kunze and et al. [50] introduce the concept of Ubiquitous Healthcare and developed a Personal Digital Assistant (PDA) as a mobile base station for communication between the monitoring device and a mobile phone through Bluetooth. Kirn raises the problem of insufficient participation of patients in treatment-related activity and introduces a www-based information platform for cancer treatments (OnkoNet Thuringia). In order to achieve better integration of patients and medical professionals in all information-related activities during diagnosis, therapy, and care, he mentioned three-level system requirements for mobile coverage of health systems in a health sector; (1) Health providers, (2) Health customers or patients and (3) Relevance of mobile computing. The key factor of these requirements is availability of health services in all parts of the health supply chain, which is promising by MHM.

Hence, in recent years, the application of mobile computing in health monitoring has increased tremendously. Mobile health monitoring can be defined as mobile computing, health information and communications technologies. This represents the evolution of computing in health systems from traditional desktop telemedicine platforms to mobile configurations [45,25,108,74,52,21,40,12,54,24]. Mobile health monitoring is a way to remotely capture health information from patients in four levels [21]:

- *level one*: Microsensors - capturing health information by using small size, intelligent low-energy active devices e.g. [25].
- *level two*: Wrist devices - monitoring health information by using combine sensors, circuits, supply, display and wireless transmission in a single box, which is very convenient for common physical activities, e.g. [108].
- *level three*: Health smart clothes - capturing information by using health sensors that have to be thin, flexible and compatible with textiles, or

made using textile technologies, such as new fibers with specific (mechanical, electrical and optical) properties [3,45,65,24,105,33,34].

- *level four*: Health smart homes - avoiding the cost and inconvenience of long hospitalization. "Exosensors" are used for measuring of the activity and behavior of patients. One of the most well-known applications for this level is continuous monitoring of patient progress in home-based treatments such as monitoring of elderly during rehabilitation and stepping treatments. In recent years, there has been an increasing trend towards the use of level four MHM in home-based treatments such as rehabilitation.

Following our discussion in Section 3.5, considering the potential benefits of using video games for encouraging patients to participate in rehabilitation treatments, mobile technology can monitor progress of patients. Mobile monitoring allows us to remotely track the treatment process on a period of time. This is one of the applications of the level four MHM.

4.4 Mobile Health Monitoring for Rehabilitation

Rehabilitation treatments often take place in four steps (see Fig 1) (1) *Referral*: The doctor refers the patient to the Occupation Therapist (OT) and informs the OT

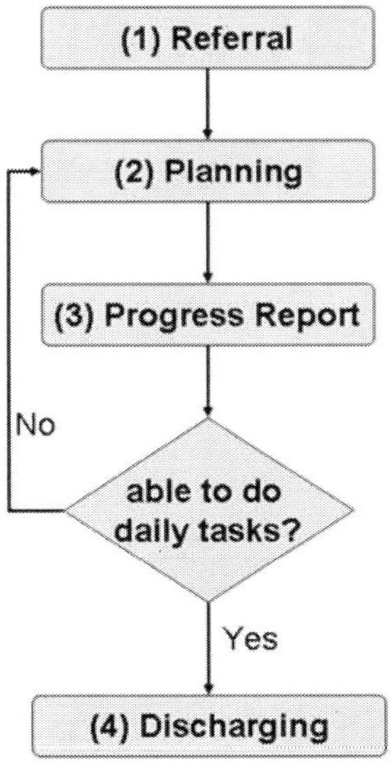

Fig. 1. Rehabilitation Treatments

about the patient's Problem. (2) *Planning*: The OT gives a rehabilitation plan to the patient. (3) *Progress Report*: The patient reports her/his progress to the OT. (4) *Discharging*: if the OT is satisfied that the patient will be able to perform daily tasks, she/he discharges the patient, otherwise the OT will go back to Step2.

This scenario will work provided the patient and the OT are located in the same place. Therefore, the OT receives direct information about the results of the patient's treatment. In home-based rehabilitation, when the patients are asked to play rehabilitation games at home, the OT unlikely receives punctual and real-time information about the game results. This affects the success of rehabilitation treatments at homes. In the next section, we propose level four of MHM to monitor Patient's progress when she/he plays a rehabilitation game at home.

One of the major questions facing the management of integrated MHM systems is how to utilize emerging Information Technology (IT) tools and techniques to facilitate cooperation between different agencies and roles involved in treatments, called cooperative roles [80]. Currently, there are different integrated standards for cooperation in distributed systems such as Internet SNMP, OSI, RM-ODP, TMN, TINA, and IETF. These standards are based on an assumption that the cooperation between roles is sufficient. Therefore, when cooperation needs to be enhanced, such as when the OT does not have access to the patient's progress in home-based rehabilitation, these standards will not be able to effectively manage to monitor patients. The major hindrance to solve this problem is the lack of a mechanism to support cooperation. We borrow the concept of contextual awareness from the field of Computer Supported Cooperative Work (CSCW) for this purpose [68,80,79,17,18].

Contextual awareness refers to the knowledge of a cooperative role based on the context. *Context* is a set of suitable states and settings concerning a user, which are relevant for a situation in the process of adapting the services and information offered to the user [20]. In stepping treatments when the patient plays rehabilitation games at home, she/he does not have sufficient cooperation with her/his OT to inform her/his progress. The patient should go to the clinic regularly, which is very inconvenient and often does not happen. As a result, the OT has a lack of contextual awareness that is caused by insufficient cooperation between the OT and the patient. Therefore, here, to have an effective mobile health monitoring system we need to enhance the cooperation by using mobile technologies.

Ray and et al [80,17,18] propose a four-step process to enhance cooperation that illustrates opportunities to share contextual information among cooperative roles. The steps are summarized as follows:

- *Step One: Recognizing the cooperative work as it is.* In this step, we analyze the actual cooperation between roles, although it may be insufficient and needs to be enhanced. Fig 2 shows the current cooperative work among Doctor, OT, and Patient in rehabilitation treatments. This cooperative work, in Fig 2, is based on the treatment process for rehabilitation presented in Fig 1.

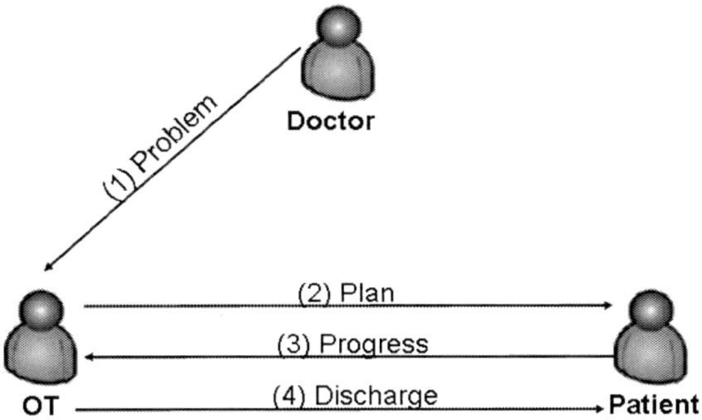

Fig. 2. Cooperative Work for Rehabilitation

- *Step Two: Recognizing Available Awareness (AA) for each Role.* In this step, we measure the cooperation by understanding of contextual awareness for each role. For different informational articles, we should find out awareness of each role. Provided the patient and the OT are located in the same place, the OT can receive direct information about the result of treatments. In home-based rehabilitation games, when the patient is at home, the OT unlikely receives punctual and on-time information about the game results (see Fig 3).

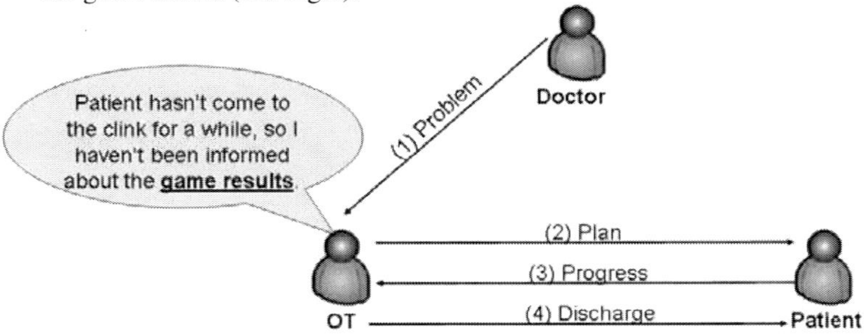

Fig. 3. Available Awareness for Rehabilitation

- *Step Three: Recognizing Required Awareness (RA) for each Role.* In this step, we find out the required knowledge of cooperative roles, which is called Required Awareness (RA), although it may be different from what actually roles are aware (AA). Fig 4 shows that the game result is required by the OT in order to continue planning or to discharge the patient.

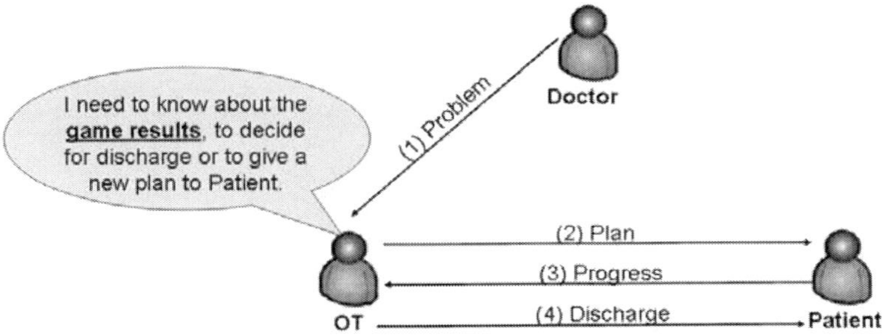

Fig. 4. Required Awareness for Rehabilitation

- *Step Four: Enhancing cooperation.* If we have such contextual information in RA that is missing in AA, then there is an opportunity to enhance cooperation among roles. This enhancement helps roles to (1) share their knowledge about missing contextual information, (2) intelligently behave when they are aware of that extra information. Step 2 and 3 illustrate that the OT is not aware of the game result as fast as it is required, which consequently shows insufficient cooperation between the OT and the patient. As such, by enhancing cooperation between the patient and the OT, (1) the patient will be able to share the game results with the OT and (2) the OT will be able to plan to continue the treatment or discharge the patient (see Fig 5).

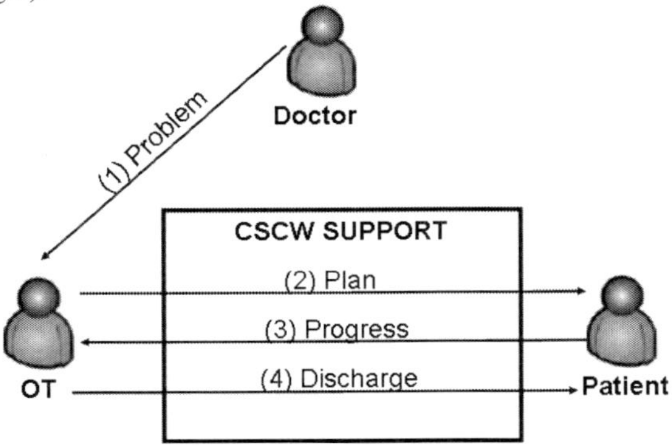

Fig. 5. CSCW Support to Enhance Cooperation between OT and Patient

Software agents are pieces of software that act on behalf of cooperative roles [71]. One of the solutions to increase awareness in cooperative environments is to take people involved and train them to act based upon awareness of their environment. However, literature [70,95] in human-computer interactions proposes use of software agents by describing different problems that can be solved with agents. Some of these problems, related to this research, are pointed out here:

- *Irrelevant information*: As we mentioned above, mobile health monitoring often needs cooperation in a highly distributed environment. Software agents can support human roles offering integrated automated cooperation to retrieve information. In order to avoid bombarding an individual with irrelevant or loosely relevant information, using software agents is beneficial [80].
- *Sporadic contacts of cooperative roles*: In mobile health monitoring, when roles need to remotely cooperate, one of the challenges is sporadic communication. Software agents, providing mediated communication among human roles, can be useful in such situations. This has been confirmed by different cases [100,107,88,78,96].

Hence, we are going to set up an agent-based architecture to enhance cooperation between the OT and the patient. Such architecture should be capable of transferring the patient's progress to the OT. It also requires providing the OT's feedback to the patient. Fig 6 presents a mobile monitoring system for home-based rehabilitation games. The designed architecture is based on interactions between human roles and software agents. Human roles i.e. Doctor, OT and Patient are represented by . In the designed monitoring system, we use two types of software agents: (1) Resident Agent [72], simply called agent, which will be installed on the game set at the Patient's home. This kind of software agent is represented by . (2) Mobile Agent, which are represented by  and will be installed onto Patient and OT's mobile phone. Fig 6 shows that mobile agents communicate together by SMS while a Bluetooth network should also be installed in the patient's home to provide communication between the Game Agent and her/his mobile (see Fig 6). In the designed system, represented in the figure, interactions and their sequences are as following: (1) the doctor refers the patient to the OT and informs the OT about the patient's problem. (2) the OT writes a SMS informing which step and how long to play for the patient (3) the OT mobile agent sends the Time-and-Step SMS to the patient mobile agent. (4) The patient mobile agent displays the Time-and-Step SMS to the patient. (5) the patient sets the game with the step and the time. Then she/he plays the game. (6) the game agent sends the number of mistakes to the patient mobile agent through bluetooth. (7) the patient mobile agent sends a SMS informing the number of mistakes. (8) the OT mobile agent displays the number-of-mistakes SMS to OT. (9) If the number is satisfactory and the OT is satisfied that the patient will be able to perform daily tasks, she/he will discharge the patient and writes the STOP SMS, otherwise the OT repeats Step2. (10) the OT mobile agent sends the STOP SMS to the patient mobile agent. (11) the patient mobile agent displays the STOP SMS to the patient.

The impact of mobile technologies for home-based treatments changes the way that health professionals traditionally deliver their services. Given a mobile health solution, the patient and health professionals will experience a radical shift in service delivery. Therefore, it is necessary to evaluate potential identified technologies, which requires an evaluation framework with customized criteria that show how the technology can be used by patients and health professionals. In the following section we present a framework to evaluate usability of such solutions as we designed here.

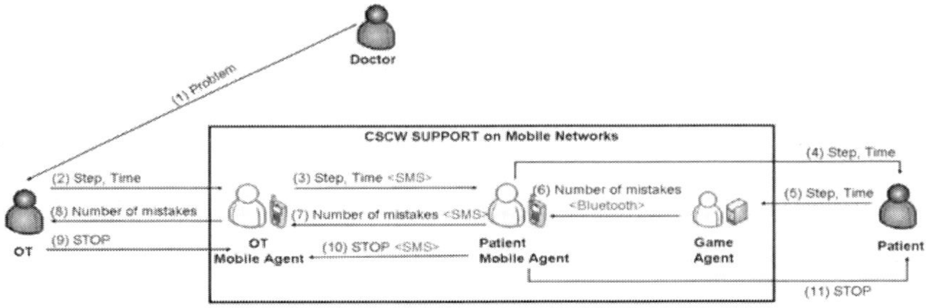

Fig. 6. Agent-based Architecture: Mobile Monitoring of Home-based Rehabilitation Games

5 Usability Evaluation Framework

Technologies are becoming more and more complicated, powerful, and mysterious, but if the systems are not practical and usable, they create problems for the user. Therefore, the operation of systems should be easy and uncomplicated to ensure maximum benefit for the user [102].

One of significant issues in designing a new technology in medical devices and introducing products to the market are social acceptance and practical usability. New technologies are very business critical and are characterized by a wide range of factors lying in the lifecycle of the product development. Therefore, American National Standards Institute's Human Factors Design Processes for Medical Devices states the usability evaluation for complying medical products [4]. Rubin [89] defines Usability Evaluation as "a process that employs participants who are representative of a particular target population to evaluate the degree to which a product or a system satisfies basic usability criteria".

The purpose of this section is to briefly describe meaning of usability and introduce a framework that we are going to use in our future imperial research for evaluating mobile monitoring of home-based rehabilitation systems. This framework is based on two well-known existing evaluation frameworks; one is for assessing usability of medical information technologies at patients' homes [47] and one is for evaluation of usability in health monitoring technologies [19].

5.1 A Framework for Usability Evaluation of Mobile Health Monitoring in Home-Based Rehabilitation Games

In order to develop a medical device and utilize the system to its full capabilities while it is facilitated by information technologies, considerations of human factor aspects in the designs of both hardware and software are vital. Therefore, Kaufman et al. [47] propose their methodological approach based on CSCW. We follow their proposed methodology that has been already applied on a home-based telemedicine system for diabetes in IDEATel project [92]. Since the concept of health monitoring has not been taken in this framework, we basically integrate this framework with the meaning of usability and guidelines for usability measurement proposed by Daniels et al. [19]. Daniels' proposal is based on internal metrics [42] and quality of product in-use [43] as it is described in ISO 9216 Quality Model.

System Description - We are going to evaluate use of our designed MHM for home-based rehabilitation games. The system involves interactions through mobile communications as it is described in Section 4.4 (see Fig 6).

Cognitive Walkthrough Evaluation - The cognitive walkthrough (CW) is, basically, a method to inspect compatibility of users' knowledge and system interface to perform a task regarding the chosen performance measurement. The method involves identifying sequences of actions and goals required to accomplish a given task by evaluating the cognitive processes of users. CW has been applied to study of usability and learnability of several distinct medical information technologies [55,75]. According to Fig 6 and considering what we discussed in Section 4.4, Table 1 describes Goals/Actions in home-based rehabilitation games.

Table 1. Goals/Actions Analysis - Cognitive Walkthrough

Goals	*Activity*
Referral	The doctor refers the patient to the OT and informs OT about the patient's problem.
Planning	1. The OT writes a SMS to the patient informing which step and how long to play. 2. The patient receives an SMS informing how long and which step she/he should play.
Progress Report	1. The patient sets the game and starts to play. 2. The OT receives a SMS informing the number of mistakes that the patient made and how long she/he played.
Discharging	1. If the results are satisfactory and the OT is satisfied that the patient is able to perform daily tasks, she/he will send a SMS discharging the patient. 2. The patient receives a SMS asking to stop the treatment.

In fact, the technology proposed for mobile monitoring is based on SMS and Bluetooth communications. These features are supported by most of available mobile phones on the market. The monitoring system does not even need Internet connection. Therefore, if the patient does not use Internet, she/he is still able to benefit from mobile monitoring while playing the rehabilitation game at home. However, according to [55], provided the patient does not oppose, we should install two cameras; one to record how the patient reacts to the system and one to record the system screen. Then we run macro and micro analysis to find out performance measures presented in Table 2. These measures are adapted from the performance measures in Daniels' framework [19] and can be measured with following two methods:

- *Macro analysis* – In order to analyse the videos recorded from patients, one of the options is Macro Analysis followed by guidelines of [55]. Macro analysis investigates performance measures for the whole system with all its functionalities and actions.
- *Micro analysis* – The next step is performance measurement for each of the actions that the patients perform. This analysis measures performance of actions one-by-one and it is adapted from [55].

Table 2. Performance *Measures* [19]

Measures
1. The time taken to complete a task
2. The number of tasks completed in a time limit
3. The ratio on successful to unsuccessful interactions
4. the number of errors
5. The time to recover from errors

Field usability evaluation - We are going to install an easy-to-use touch screen and ask five different categories of questions. The field usability evaluation is part of the Kaufman's framework, although the categories have been borrowed from Daniels' framework [19]. Therefore, the meaning of usability is for monitoring systems, although the field usability evaluation is based on what has been proposed for home-based medical devices.

- *Thinking aloud* – This method is one of the most successful methods to evaluate how users think and not only what they do [93]. This method has been recognised as one of the most successful methods in evaluation of usability of electronic medical devices [22,55]. The idea is a free comment area in the touch screen that can be filled by patients when they use the system. Then, we will classify and code the comments using supportive tools such as those introduced in [22,89].
- *Question asking method* – We will develop electronic questionnaires which will appear on the touch screen. The nature of this method is similar to the think-aloud method, but the goal is investigating how the system works from Patient's point of view. Therefore, we just select those actions in Table 1 that are being performed by patients. We have designed our questions (see Table 3).
- *Interviews* - Some aspects of usability can be found from the OT's point of view by simply asking how they feel about the system under study, how the system can help them and their clinics and what recommendations should be taken into account. However, such a study requires caution, especially in interpreting the OTs' opinions [86].

Table 3. Questions for Question Asking Method

Activity	*Questions*
Patient receives a SMS informing how long and which step she/he should play.	1. Do you know which step and how long you should play? Yes ( ) No ( ) 2. Do you like this feature to receive your plan by SMSs? Yes ( ) No ( ) 3. How would you rate the ease of use of the product? Very difficult ( ) Difficult ( ) Affordable ( ) Easy ( )
Patient sets the game and starts to play.	1. Do you know how to set the game? Yes ( ) No ( ) 2. Do you like the set up wizard? Yes ( ) No ( ) 3. How would you rate the ease of use of the product? Very difficult ( ) Difficult ( ) Affordable ( ) Easy ( )
Patient receives a SMS asking to stop playing.	Do you like this feature to receive your discharge by SMSs? Yes ( ) No ( ).
General interest question	1. Would you buy his product if it is available in the market? Yes ( ) No ( ) Maybe ( ) 2. Do you think this system will help you to get a quicker response, if an incident happens while you play the game? Yes ( ) No ( ) Maybe ( )

6 Conclusion and Future Work

This chapter after a brief introduction on Games for Health, specifically rehabilitation treatments, shows that rehabilitation research reports that exercises, designed for physical therapy, are often dull and repetitive. Therefore, adherence to training is poor [26], which can be improved by involving patients in interactive games [15,87,26]. There are also bodies of research that show home-based rehabilitation, providing convenience to patients, are more effective than traditional methods [97,94,49]. However, there is an empirical report that shows the role of monitoring in home-based rehabilitation has been largely ignored [82]. The report shows that hospital-based rehabilitation treatments are more effective than unsupervised home-based rehabilitation exercises. This chapter has proposed a mobile monitoring system to address the supervision problem of home-based rehabilitation games.

The idea of bringing rehabilitation treatments to homes requires supervision and reviewing of patients' progress. Without using mobile technology, patients report their progress time-by-time, which is often not enough for an effective treatment. Therefore mobile monitoring allows patients to easily transfer their accrued progress after each exercise to her/his OT. This increases the OT's awareness of the patient's progress and accordingly improves the efficacy of rehabilitation treatments. In order to achieve maximum usability, we have chosen very basic technologies i.e. SMS and Bluetooth that are supported by most of the mobile phones.

The proposed MHM is new and untried either in a simulated or real production environment. An initial proof of concept as an exemplar is made in the chapter while exemplars are a common way to provide initial validation to a new method in software engineering. We are also planning to run an experiment based on a usability evaluation framework described in Section 5.

The nature of the rehabilitation game is such that it may be possible for a patient to suffer a fall while one of the benefits of monitoring is fall detection. In this case, the system should detect the incident and bring online a hierarchy of recovery services. This can start with sending an alarm to the hospital. In order to achieve this goal, fall detection requires monitoring sensors attached to the patient's body. Although, currently, the proposed system does not support such a feature, we are planning to add sensing devices with bluetooth communication with the patient's mobile phone. Therefore, the system will also be able to detect falls and alarm emergency and recovery services. Furthermore, fall detection ensures patients that they are under monitoring and if an incident happens, they will be safe. This will help to increase the usability acceptance of the system.

References

1. Albert, A.: R. Virtual Reality and Cognitive Rehabilitation: A Brief Review. The Journal of Head Trauma Rehabilitation 12(6) (1997)
2. Anderson, C.A., Bushman, B.J.: Effects of violent video games on aggressive behavior, aggressive cognition, aggressive affect, physiological arousal, and prosocial behavior: a meta-analytic review of the scientific literature. Psychological Science: A Journal of the American Psychological Society / APS 12(5), 353–359 (2001)

3. Anliker, U., Ward, J.A., Lukowicz, P., et al.: AMON: a wearable multiparameter medical monitoring and alert system. IEEE Transactions on Information Technology in Biomedicine: A Publication of the IEEE Engineering in Medicine and Biology Society 8(4), 415–427 (2004)
4. ANSI/AAMI. Human Factors Design Process for Medical Devices. Association for the Advancement of Medical Instrumentation (2001)
5. Atchison, B., Dirette, D.K.: Conditions in occupational therapy. Lippincott Williams & Wilkins (2007)
6. Beale, I.L., Kato, P.M., Marin-Bowling, V.M., Guthrie, N., Cole, S.W.: Improvement in cancer-related knowledge following use of a psychoeducational video game for adolescents and young adults with cancer. The Journal of Adolescent Health: Official Publication of the Society for Adolescent Medicine 41(3), 263–270 (2007)
7. Bergeron, B.P.: Learning & retention in adaptive serious games. Studies in Health Technology and Informatics 132, 26–30 (2008)
8. Bhangu, A., Lwin, M., Dias, R.: Wimbledon or bust: Nintendo Wii related rupture of the extensor pollicis longus tendon. The Journal of Hand Surgery, European 34(3), 399–400 (2009)
9. Borges, M., Brezillon, P., Pino, J., Pomerol, J.: Bringing context to CSCW. In: The Proceedings of The 8th International Conference on Computer Supported Cooperative Work in Design, vol. 2, pp. 161–166 (2004)
10. Case-Smith, J.: Occupational Therapy for Children. C.V. Mosby (2000)
11. Chan, L., Beaver, S., MacLehose, R.F., Jha, A., Maciejewski, M., Doctor, J.N.: Disability and health care costs in the Medicare population. Archives of Physical Medicine and Rehabilitation 83(9), 1196–1201 (2002)
12. Cheng, P., Tsai, L., Lu, L., Yang, D.: The Design of PDA-Based Biomedical Data Processing and Analysis for Intelligent Wearable Health Monitoring Systems. In: Proceedings of the The Fourth International Conference on Computer and Information Technology, pp. 879–884. IEEE Computer Society, Los Alamitos (2004)
13. Christiansen, C., Abreu, B., Ottenbacher, K., Huffman, K., Masel, B., Culpepper, R.: Task performance in virtual environments used for cognitive rehabilitation after traumatic brain injury. Archives of Physical Medicine and Rehabilitation 79(8), 888–892 (1998)
14. Chuang, Y.: Massively multiplayer online role-playing game-induced seizures: a neglected health problem in Internet addiction. Cyberpsychology & Behavior: The Impact of the Internet, Multimedia and Virtual Reality on Behavior and Society 9(4), 451–456 (2006)
15. Colombo, R., Pisano, F., Mazzone, A., et al.: Design strategies to improve patient motivation during robot-aided rehabilitation. Journal of NeuroEngineering and Rehabilitation 4, 3 (2007)
16. Daley, E.: Wireless interoperability. Public Manage 85(4), 6–10 (2003)
17. Daneshgar, F., Ray, P.: Awareness modelling and its application in cooperative network management. In: Proceedings of the Seventh International Conference on Parallel and Distributed Systems, pp. 357–363 (2000)
18. Daneshgar, F., Bunker, D., Lee, K.M.: Identifying opportunities for enhancing collaboration in the Australian health insurance sector. International Journal of Business Process Integration and Management 1(3), 210–218 (2006)

19. Daniels, J., Fels, S., Kushniruk, A., Lim, J., Ansermino, J.: A framework for evaluating usability of clinical monitoring technology. Journal of Clinical Monitoring and Computing 21(5), 323–330 (2007)
20. Dey, A.K.: Understanding and Using Context. Personal Ubiquitous Comput. 5(1), 4–7 (2001)
21. Dittmar, A., Axisa, F., Delhomme, G., Gehin, C.: New concepts and technologies in home care and ambulatory monitoring. Studies in Health Technology and Informatics 108, 9–35 (2004)
22. Dumas, J.S., Redish, J.: A practical guide to usability testing. Intellect Books, Bristol (1999)
23. Duque, G., Fung, S., Mallet, L., Posel, N., Fleiszer, D.: Learning while having fun: the use of video gaming to teach geriatric house calls to medical students. Journal of the American Geriatrics Society 56(7), 1328–1332 (2008)
24. European Research in IS World. WEALTHY - Wearable Health Care System (2002), `http://www.ist-world.org/ProjectDetails.aspx?ProjectId=0d9029df6a0d4e8d9d478c26fa1b7233&SourceDatabaseId=9cd97ac2e51045e39c2ad6b86dce1ac2`
25. Fensli, R., Gunnarson, E., Hejlesen, O.: A wireless ECG system for continuous event recording and communication to a clinical alarm station. In: 26th Annual International Conference of the IEEE, Engineering in Medicine and Biology Society IEMBS 2004, pp. 2208–2211 (2004)
26. Flores, E., Tobon, G., Cavallaro, E., Cavallaro, F.I., Perry, J.C., Keller, T.: Improving patient motivation in game development for motor deficit rehabilitation. In: Proceedings of the 2008 International Conference on Advances in Computer Entertainment Technology, pp. 381–384. ACM, New York (2008)
27. Frost & Sullivan Research Service: European Markets for Healthcare IT Platforms. Frost & Sullivan Research Service (2007)
28. Gentile, D.A., Anderson, C.A., Yukawa, S., et al.: The effects of prosocial video games on prosocial behaviors: international evidence from correlational, longitudinal, and experimental studies. Personality and Social Psychology Bulletin 35(6), 752–763 (2009)
29. Graf, D.L., Pratt, L.V., Hester, C.N., Short, K.R.: Playing active video games increases energy expenditure in children. Pediatrics 124(2), 534–540 (2009)
30. Grealy, M.A., Johnson, D.A., Rushton, S.K.: Improving cognitive function after brain injury: the use of exercise and virtual reality. Archives of Physical Medicine and Rehabilitation 80(6), 661–667 (1999)
31. Grüsser, S.M., Thalemann, R., Griffiths, M.D.: Excessive computer game playing: evidence for addiction and aggression? Cyberpsychology & Behavior: The Impact of the Internet, Multimedia and Virtual Reality on Behavior and Society 10(2), 290–292 (2007)
32. Gwinup, G., Haw, T., Elias, A.: Cardiovascular changes in video-game players. Cause for concern? Postgraduate Medicine 74(6), 245–248 (1983)
33. van Halteren, A., Bults, R., Wac, K., et al.: Wireless body area networks for healthcare: the MobiHealth project. Studies in Health Technology and Informatics 108, 181–193 (2004)
34. Hao, Y., Foster, R.: Wireless body sensor networks for health-monitoring applications. Physiological Measurement 29(11), R27–R56 (2008)

35. Hardy, L.L., Dobbins, T.A., Denney-Wilson, E.A., Okely, A.D., Booth, M.L.: Sedentariness, small-screen recreation, and fitness in youth. American Journal of Preventive Medicine 36(2), 120–125 (2009)
36. Haugeneder, H., Steiner, D.: Multi-agent cooperation — Concepts and applications. In: Design and Implementation of Symbolic Computation Systems, pp. 195–197 (1996)
37. Higgins, S.: Motor Skill Acquisition. Phys. Ther. 71(2), 123–139 (1991)
38. Hoffman, H.G., Doctor, J.N., Patterson, D.R., Carrougher, G.J., Furness, T.A.: Virtual reality as an adjunctive pain control during burn wound care in adolescent patients. Pain 85(1-2), 305–309 (2000)
39. Holden, M., Todorov, E.: Use of Virtual Environments in Motor Learning and Rehabilitation. In: Handbook of Virtual Environments: Design, Implementation, and Applications. Lawrence Elbraum Associates, Mahwah (2002)
40. Husemann, D., Narayanaswa, C., Nidd, M.: Personal Mobile Hub. In: Proceedings of the Eighth International Symposium on Wearable Computers, pp. 85–91. IEEE Computer Society, Los Alamitos (2004)
41. IDC Research: China Healthcare Industry IT Solution 2008–2012 Forecast and Analysis. IDC Research, China (2008)
42. IHS: ISO TR 9126-3 Software Engineering - Product Quality - Part 3: Internal Metrics. International Organization for Standardization (2003)
43. IHS: ISO TR 9126-4 Software engineering Product quality Part 4: Quality in use metrics. International Organization for Standardization (2004)
44. Jack, D., Boian, R., Merians, A.S., et al.: Virtual reality-enhanced stroke rehabilitation. IEEE Transactions on Neural Systems and Rehabilitation Engineering: A Publication of the IEEE Engineering in Medicine and Biology Society 9(3), 308–318 (2001)
45. Jovanov, E., Milenkovic, A., Otto, C., de Groen, P.: A wireless body area network of intelligent motion sensors for computer assisted physical rehabilitation. Journal of Neuroengineering and Rehabilitation 2(1), 6 (2005)
46. Hammell, K.W.: Spinal cord injury rehabilitation. Chapman & Hall, London (1995)
47. Kaufman, D.R., Patel, V.L., Hilliman, C., et al.: Usability in the real world: assessing medical information technologies in patients' homes. Journal of Biomedical Informatics 36(1-2), 45–60 (2003)
48. Keith, R.A., Granger, C.V., Hamilton, B.B., Sherwin, F.S.: The functional independence measure: a new tool for rehabilitation. Advances in Clinical Rehabilitation 1, 6–18 (1987)
49. Khuzadi, M.: On Health Monitoring. In: Aerospace Conference, pp. 1–8. IEEE, Los Alamitos (2008)
50. Kirn, S.: Ubiquitous Healthcare: The OnkoNet Mobile Agents Architecture. In: Objects, Components, Architectures, Services, and Applications for a Networked World, pp. 265–277 (2003)
51. Kizony, R., Raz, L., Katz, N., Weingarden, H., Weiss, P.L.T.: Video-capture virtual reality system for patients with paraplegic spinal cord injury. Journal of Rehabilitation Research and Development 42(5), 595–608 (2005)
52. Konstantas, D., van Halteren, A., Bults, R., et al.: Mobile patient monitoring: the MobiHealth system. Studies in Health Technology and Informatics 103, 307–314 (2004)

53. Krause, J.S., Kemp, B., Coker, J.: Depression after spinal cord injury: Relation to gender, ethnicity, aging, and socioeconomic indicators. Archives of Physical Medicine and Rehabilitation 81(8), 1099–1109 (2000)
54. Kumar, S., Kambhatla, K., Hu, F., Lifson, M., Xiao, Y.: Ubiquitous computing for remote cardiac patient monitoring: a survey. Int. J. Telemedicine Appl., 1–19 (2008)
55. Kushniruk, A.W., Kaufman, D.R., Patel, V.L., Lévesque, Y., Lottin, P.: Assessment of a computerized patient record system: a cognitive approach to evaluating medical technology. M.D. Computing: Computers in Medical Practice 13(5), 406–415 (1996)
56. Lenze, E.J., Munin, M.C., Quear, T., et al.: Significance of poor patient participation in physical and occupational therapy for functional outcome and length of stay. Archives of Physical Medicine and Rehabilitation 85(10), 1599–1601 (2004)
57. Lenze, E.J., Munin, M.C., Quear, T., et al.: The Pittsburgh Rehabilitation Participation Scale: reliability and validity of a clinician-rated measure of participation in acute rehabilitation. Archives of Physical Medicine and Rehabilitation 85(3), 380–384 (2004)
58. Lieberman, D.A.: Management of chronic pediatric diseases with interactive health games: theory and research findings. The Journal of Ambulatory Care Management 24(1), 26–38 (2001)
59. Mackay, J., Mensah, G.: The Atlas of Heart Disease and Stroke. World Health Organization (2004)
60. Maclean, N., Pound, P.: A critical review of the concept of patient motivation in the literature on physical rehabilitation. Soc. Sci. Med. 50(4), 495–506 (2000)
61. Magrabi, F., Lovell, N., Henry, R., Celler, B.: Development and Evaluation of a Web-based System for Home Monitoring in Cystic Fibrosis. In: The Proceedings of Health Informatics Conference (HIC 2000), pp. 301–306 (2000)
62. Malkary, G.: Healthcare Without Bounds: Trends in Mobile Communications. Spyglass Consulting Group (2006)
63. Maloney, A.E., Bethea, T.C., Kelsey, K.S., et al.: A pilot of a video game (DDR) to promote physical activity and decrease sedentary screen time. Obesity (Silver Spring, Md.) 16(9), 2074–2080 (2008)
64. MarketsandMarkets: Global Healthcare Information Technology (2009 - 2014). MarketsandMarkets (2009)
65. Martin, T., Jovanov, E., Raskovic, D.: Issues in Wearable Computing for Medical Monitoring Applications: A Case Study of a Wearable ECG Monitoring Device. In: Proceedings of the 4th IEEE International Symposium on Wearable Computers, p. 43. IEEE Computer Society, Los Alamitos (2000)
66. Mathers, C.D., Vos, E.T., Stevenson, C.E., Begg, S.J.: The burden of disease and injury in Australia. Bulletin of the World Health Organization 79(11), 1076–1084 (2001)
67. Merians, A.S., Poizner, H., Boian, R., Burdea, G., Adamovich, S.: Sensorimotor training in a virtual reality environment: does it improve functional recovery poststroke? Neurorehabilitation and Neural Repair 20(2), 252–267 (2006)
68. Mynatt, E.: Computer Supported Cooperative Work (1999), `http://www.cc.gatech.edu/gvu/cscw/`
69. Nash, E.B., Edwards, G.W., Thompson, J.A., Barfield, W.: A Review of Presence and Performance in Virtual Environments. International Journal of Human-Computer Interaction 12(1), 1 (2000)
70. Nwana, H.S., Nduma, D.T.: A Perspective on Software Agents Research (1999)

71. Nwana, H.S., Azarmi, N. (eds.): Software Agents and Soft Computing: Towards Enhancing Machine Intelligence, Concepts and Applications. Springer, Heidelberg (1997)
72. O'Donoghue, J.M.: Context-Sensitive Quality Data Management for Pervasive Computing Environments (2007), `http://www.computing.dcu.ie/research/dataquality/thesis/thesis/John.ODonoghue.pdf`
73. O'Connor, R.J., Murray, P.C.: Review of spinal cord injuries in Ireland. Spinal Cord: The Official Journal of the International Medical Society of Paraplegia 44(7), 445–448 (2006)
74. Oliver, N., Flores-Mangas, F.: HealthGear: a real-time wearable system for monitoring and analyzing physiological signals. In: International Workshop on Wearable and Implantable Body Sensor Networks, BSN 2006, vol. 4, p. 64 (2006)
75. Patel, V.L., Kaufman, D.R.: Medical informatics and the science of cognition. Journal of the American Medical Informatics Association: JAMIA 5(6), 493–502 (1998)
76. Peek, A.C., Ibrahim, T., Abunasra, H., Waller, D., Natarajan, R.: White-out from a Wii: traumatic haemothorax sustained playing Nintendo Wii. Annals of the Royal College of Surgeons of England 90(6), W9–W10 (2008)
77. Peng, W.: Design and evaluation of a computer game to promote a healthy diet for young adults. Health Communication 24(2), 115–127 (2009)
78. Ray, P., Paramesh, N.: Multi-agent service infrastructure for cooperative management. In: Global Telecommunications Conference on GLOBECOM 2002, pp. 2999–3003. IEEE, Los Alamitos (2002)
79. Ray, P., Parameswaran, N., Chan, V., Yu, W.: Awareness modelling in collaborative mobile e-health. J. Telemed Telecare 14(7), 381–385 (2008)
80. Ray, P., Shahrestani, S.A., Daneshgar, F.: The Role of Fuzzy Awareness Modelling in Cooperative Management. Information Systems Frontiers 7(3), 299–316 (2005)
81. Rebeiro, K.L., Cook, J.V.: Opportunity, not prescription: an exploratory study of the experience of occupational engagement. Canadian Journal of Occupational Therapy. Revue Canadienne D'ergothérapie 66(4), 176–187 (1999)
82. Regensteiner, J.G., Meyer, T.J., Krupski, W.C., Cranford, L.S., Hiatt, W.R., Regensteiner, J.G.: Hospital vs Home-Based Exercise Rehabilitation for Patients with Peripheral Arterial Occlusive Disease. Angiology 48(4), 291–300 (1997)
83. Reid, P.P., Compton, W.D., Grossman, J.H., et al.: Building a Better Delivery System (2005)
84. Robinson, R.J., Barron, D.A., Grainger, A.J., Venkatesh, R.: Wii knee. Emergency Radiology 15(4), 255–257 (2008)
85. Rodin, G., Voshart, K.: Depression in the medically ill: an overview. The American Journal of Psychiatry 143(6), 696–705 (1986)
86. Root, R.W., Draper, S.: Questionnaires as a software evaluation tool. In: Proceedings of the SIGCHI conference on Human Factors in Computing Systems, pp. 83–87. ACM, New York (1983)
87. Rosser, J.C., Lynch, P.J., Cuddihy, L., Gentile, D.A., Klonsky, J., Merrell, R.: The impact of video games on training surgeons in the 21st century. Archives of Surgery (Chicago, Ill.: 1960) 142(2), 181–186 (2007) (discusssion 186)
88. Rousseau, D., Moulin, B.: Mixed Initiative in Interactions between Software Agents. In: Proc. 1997 Spring Symposium On Computer Models For Mixed Initiative Interaction. AAAI Press, Menlo (1997)

89. Rubin, J.: Handbook of Usability Testing: How to Plan, Design, and Conduct Effective Tests. Wiley, Chichester (1994)
90. Sanchez-Vives, M.V., Slater, M.: From presence to consciousness through virtual reality. Nature Reviews. Neuroscience 6(4), 332–339 (2005)
91. Schwaibold, M., Gmelin, M., Wagner, G.V., Schöchlin, J., Bolz, A.: Key factors for personal health monitoring and diagnosis device. In: Mobile Computing in Medicine, Second Conference on Mobile Computing in Medicine, Workshop of the Project Group MoCoMed, GMDS-Fachbereich Medizinische Informatik & GI-Fachausschuss 4.7, GI, pp. 143–150 (2002)
92. Shea, S., Starren, J., Weinstock, R.S., et al.: Columbia University's Informatics for Diabetes Education and Telemedicine (IDEATel) Project: Rationale and Design. J. Am. Med. Inform. Assoc. 9(1), 49–62 (2002)
93. Someren, M.W.V., Barnard, Y.F., Sandberg, J.A.C.: The Think Aloud Method: A Practical Guide to Modelling Cognitive Processes. Academic Press, London (1994)
94. Suttie, A.: Care home residents use Nintendo Wii to relive their sporting days. Community Care (2009), `http://www.communitycare.co.uk/Articles/2009/03/03/110886/care-home-residents-use-nintendo-wii-to-relive-their-sporting.html`
95. Taurisson, N., Tchounikine, P.: Mixing human and software agents: a case study. In: Proceedings of The 3rd IEEE International Conference on Advanced Learning Technologies, pp. 239–243 (2003)
96. Taurisson, N., Tchounikine, P.: Mixing human and software agents: a case study. In: Proceedings of The 3rd IEEE International Conference on Advanced Learning Technologies, pp. 239–243 (2003)
97. Tinetti, M.E., Baker, D.I., Gottschalk, M., et al.: Home-based multicomponent rehabilitation program for older persons after hip fracture: a randomized trial. Archives of Physical Medicine and Rehabilitation 80(8), 916–922 (1999)
98. Trombly, C.A.: Occupation: purposefulness and meaningfulness as therapeutic mechanisms. 1995 Eleanor Clarke Slagle Lecture. The American Journal of Occupational Therapy.: Official Publication of the American Occupational Therapy Association 49(10), 960–972 (1995)
99. Trombly, C.A., Radomski, M.V.: Occupational Therapy for Physical Dysfunction. Lippincott Williams & Wilkins (2001)
100. Ulieru, M., Doursat, R.: Emergent Engineering:A Radical Paradigm Shift. International Journal of Autonomous and Adaptive Communications Systems (2009)
101. Vincent, C., Deaudelin, I., Robichaud, L., et al.: Rehabilitation needs for older adults with stroke living at home: perceptions of four populations. BMC Geriatrics 7, 20 (2007)
102. Wang, E.M.: Usability evaluation for human-computer interaction, HCI (1992)
103. Warburton, D.E.R., Bredin, S.S.D., Horita, L.T.L., et al.: The health benefits of interactive video game exercise. Applied Physiology, Nutrition, and Metabolism = Physiologie Appliquée, Nutrition Et Métabolisme 32(4), 655–663 (2007)
104. Windich-Biermeier, A., Sjoberg, I., Dale, J.C., Eshelman, D., Guzzetta, C.E.: Effects of distraction on pain, fear, and distress during venous port access and venipuncture in children and adolescents with cancer. Journal of Pediatric Oncology Nursing: Official Journal of the Association of Pediatric Oncology Nurses 24(1), 8–19 (2007)

105. Winters, J.M., Wang, Y., Winters, J.M.: Wearable sensors and telerehabilitation. IEEE Engineering in Medicine and Biology Magazine: The Quarterly Magazine of the Engineering in Medicine & Biology Society 22(3), 56–65 (2003)
106. Wood, D.J.: The "How!" sign–a central palmar blister induced by overplaying on a Nintendo console. Archives of Disease in Childhood 84(4), 288 (2001)
107. Yuan, Y., Detlor, B.: Intelligent mobile crisis response systems. Commun. ACM 48(2), 95–98 (2005)
108. Yuan-Hsiang, L., I-Chien, J., Ko, P., Chen, Y.-Y., Wong, J.-M., Jan, G.-J.: A wireless PDA-based physiological monitoring system for patient transport. IEEE Transactions on Information Technology in Biomedicine 8(4), 439–447 (2004)

Chapter 8
Intelligent Decision-Support in Virtual Reality Healthcare and Rehabilitation

A.L. Brooks

Esbjerg Technical Institute, Aalborg University, SensoramaLab,
Niels Bohrs vej 8, 6700 Esbjerg, Denmark
anthony.lewis.brooks@gmail.com
tb@create.aau.dk

Abstract. Intelligent Decision-Support (IDS) mechanisms to improve an 'in-action' facilitator intervention model and 'on-action' evaluation and refinement model are proposed for contemporary Virtual Reality Healthcare & Rehabilitation training. The 'Zone of Optimized Motivation' (ZOOM) model and the 'Hermeneutic Action Research Recursive Reflection' model have emerged from a body of virtual reality research called SoundScapes. The work targets all ages and all abilities through gesture-control of responsive multimedia within Virtual Interactive Space (VIS). VIS is an interactive information environment at the core of an open-ended custom system where unencumbered residual function manipulates selected audiovisual and robotic feedback that results in afferent-efferent neural feedback loop closure. Such loop closure is hypothesized as the reason why such interactive system environments are so effective in the context of rehabilitation and healthcare. The approach is adaptive across the range of dysfunction, from the most profoundly disabled to traditionally developed. This proposal considers enhancing VIS data exchange, i.e. human input information matched to responsive content, through dynamic decision-support of adjustment of difficulty encountered. To date facilitator role has included manual parameter manipulation of interface to affect an invisible active zone quality (typically, sensitivity or location) and/or content quality. In-action human adjustment-decisions are according to interpretation of user state and engagement. Questioned is whether automated support for such decisions is feasible so that dynamic difficulty adjustment (DDA) of that which is encountered by the user is considered optimal to goal. Core issues are presented to detail and justify the concept. Findings are related to current trends with conclusions reflecting on potential impact.

Keywords: Afferent-Efferent Neural Feedback Loop Closure, Gesture-control, Sensor-based Interactivity, Virtual Reality Healthcare & Rehabilitation, Virtual Interactive Space (VIS), Dynamic Difficulty Adjustment (DDA).

1 Introduction

This position chapter discusses a body of research that originated from a teenager's simple interactions with a profoundly disabled uncle. Empowerment

S. Brahnam & L.C. Jain (Eds.): Adv. Comput. Intell. Paradigms in Healthcare 5, SCI 326, pp. 143–169.
springerlink.com

was through adaptive use of a traditional foot pedal device normally used by a guitarist to control musical parameters. Manipulation of auditory feedback was via upper torso gesture that raised or lowered the pedal positioned under an elbow. Euphoric response and continued, motivated interactions followed with resulting life quality change and well-being alongside improved communications and social interactions by the disabled uncle.

The profound impact and understanding of potentials from empowering leisure, recreation and entertainment as fun training through sensing technologies and responsive multimedia were not realized until a decade and a half later. A hybrid electro-acoustic instrument to empower disabled people to be able to creatively express and freely play with sounds through residual gesture was realized. Subsequent studies explored beyond solely auditory. Motion controlled audiovisuals and robotic devices was also explored as feedback stimulus.

To date, abductively-generated models have evolved from SoundScapes' applied research. These models focus on how (1) facilitator intervention optimizes motivated-participation in technology-enhanced therapeutic training sessions, and (2) how original session material is analyzed and reanalyzed recursively to optimize knowledge and knowing. Each model is presented in this position chapter.

Sessions using this form of 'training' differ from traditional rehabilitation intervention as fun user-experiences are targeted via gesture-control of virtual reality (games or abstract content in the form of digital painting or music making). Thus, a whole person-approach rather than a traditional therapist approach to intervention underpins the work – this is described elsewhere in this chapter.

A hypothesis is that intelligent decision-support in the form of machine-learning can be developed to improve such intervention that has a goal of life quality. This position hypothesis is posited in this chapter.

The next section outlines the original apparatus and method that evolved from the research to be responsible for a patent [10] on how gesture-responsive non-intrusive sensor-based interactive multimedia can be used in non-formal healthcare rehabilitation, and education. A background section then follows which informs how performance art has been influential in development of the concept.

1.1 Outline

A prototype open-ended interactive multimedia system was created to investigate a discovered need of how people with profound disability, who for example cannot hold a traditional musical instrument, paint brush or computer mouse, desire to express themselves creatively and playfully just as others of higher function are able to.

To enable access to such expressivity, the system utilizes whatever residual physical function is available to generate data via movement within active sensor spaces. Generated data controls multimedia.

This player space is central to the interactive virtual environment referred to as Virtual Interactive Space (VIS)[7].

The invisible space that acts as the human interface to the open-ended system is flexible in that it can be volumetric/3D, linear, or planar according to technology used (figure 1). The technologies can also be mixed and matched to suit each case.

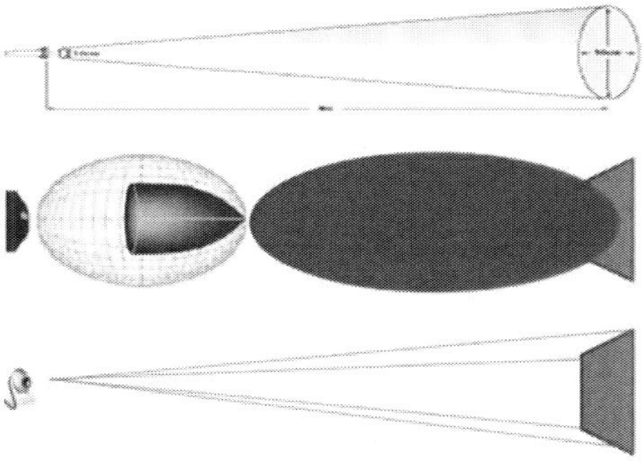

Fig. 1. Non-invasive sensor profiles used in SoundScapes

The sensors are non-invasive to enable data-generation from unencumbered motion, i.e. no need to wear, hold or touch any input device. The unencumbered gesture controls responsive multimedia that is pleasing, direct and immediate so as to digitally mirror input to stimulate the user to further react intuitively in such a way as to become immersed in the interaction. Motivation is augmented. The mirroring technique reinforces a participant's awareness of movement and proprioception and is developed from observations of traditional silver mirror use at rehabilitation institutes to train profoundly disabled.

Aesthetic Resonance (AR) [11] is targeted as exhibited user state via the mirroring technique. This is achieved from an optimized session set-up and experienced facilitator intervention. In such a set-up, mediating technology affordances influence a user's sense of self-agency leading to empowerment and potential microdevelopment. The aesthetic value relates to how the user recognizes associations between input physical action/motion and the abstract feedback that stimulates further action. Resonance is a known quality of the motor system in how it responds during observation of an action [47]. This form of resonance behavior links directly to the human condition, and the body's capacity for 'release phenomena' [57] and 'response facilitation' [12]. Related resonance is where higher order motor action plans are coded so that an internal copying of the observed action - in this case the multimedia response; is not repeated but is rather used as the basis for a next action [47]. In this way Aesthetic Resonance associates directly to closure of the afferent-efferent neural feedback loop, which is suggested as a reason why interactive multimedia is so effective within rehabilitation training [11].

The next section introduces the background of the work.

1.2 Background

The patent [10] resulted from the author's research which began around 1985. The concepts and approaches in SoundScapes evolved from an engineering education, artistic background (e.g., early work shown at The Institute of Contemporary Arts

(ICA), London around 1975), and close association with severely disabled family members.

Over the years, SoundScapes has been used in the author's own stage productions and performances, interactive installations (e.g., in Museums of Modern Art, international commissions), and as a therapeutic supplement in healthcare and rehabilitation. It is the latter that is in focus of this chapter, however linkages to performance art should be evident to those in the field.

The research explores alternative means of creative expression and focuses on invisible collection of body function signal data.

Since the research beginnings, systems to explore the concept have been created with a variety of mediums, i.e., arrays of input motion sensing devices mapped to an assortment of (output) multimodal contents. These have led to the current open conglomeration where hardware and software are mixed and matched appropriate to the user.

User groups

Attention for the therapeutic work has been to users who are profoundly disabled. This is a community consisting of many who are unable to speak, yet, through their idiosyncratic means, are able to communicate to guide facilitator intervention. Intervention in this case refers to the actions taken by the facilitator in training sessions.

Much has been learnt from such sessions with extreme cases where the author has had the role as facilitator and designer working with therapists and healthcare workers that usually know the user well. Such learning has contributed to the system, conception and methodology resulting in it being successfully applied within other sectors of disability with people having higher functions. These include acquired brain injury (stroke), Down syndrome, Cerebral Palsy, and many others. Increased use is also in the growing sector of aged towards supplementing future service needs.

Recent adoptions by healthcare and rehabilitation professionals of affordable commercially available game systems, such as Nintendo Wii, correlate to the author's original concept. Such contemporary game platforms utilizing alternative sensor-based gesture-controllers improve upon the author's basic gesture-controlled interactive non-abstract content, i.e. video games. These have been used in SoundScapes' therapeutic situations since around 1998.

An example of game-based intervention is where the Sony EyeToy was used in a study designed and led by the author involving children (n=18) at two hospitals in Denmark and Sweden. The children, 10 females and 8 males, were of high function and across the age range of 5-12 years-of-age, (mean 7.66). Control was those not in sessions.

The children's gesture controlled screen artifacts which motivated further interaction and physical activity [9]. Doctors and play therapists who conducted the clinic sessions responded favorably to children's reactions. However, in this investigation the design was that there was no opportunity given for the facilitator(s) to change game parameters. Thus, those with high competence quickly became bored. Equating to the state of flow [15, 16, and 17] being diminished. A need was for parameter programming change of both human motion data capture device (i.e. feedforward) and presented content, i.e. visuals, audio, (i.e. feedback). Addressing this need in a high-quality game is unusual, yet, it would give opportunities for facilitators to adapt the situation to maintain user engagement and motivation.

Differing from this example is a SoundScapes study with learning challenged individuals at a school for cultural education and at a special school for youngsters who are profoundly disabled [8].

The open-ended system enabled programming of both feedforward and feedback that enabled facilitator parameter change to motivate the users in an optimal way. This is often done on the fly in response to user interaction with the mediating technology.

Reflecting this need for an open-ended system and approach this chapter presents the models that support the decisions in sessions as well as suggesting the related next step to further the work through machine-supported decision-making to support the service personnel load of the future. Machine-supported decision-making is seen as a means to optimize calibration and adaptation of the interface in 'real-time' that is matched to the content control.

The next section briefly introduces the concept and open system conglomerations including the focused system that was created to be adaptive to individual needs and preferences. The facilitator role is presented in the subsequent section followed by a section on in-action and on-action decision-making.

2 Concept Need and System Conglomerations

Population demographics are changing dramatically so that aged and disabled are predicted to increase at an astounding rate. The concept in question was designed to be open and without constraint of user ability or age. It has been subject of research and development since the mid-nineteen eighties and application is reported in numerous articles. It has evolved through experimentation and prototype iterations via system conglomerations consisting of libraries of input device and output content that can be mixed and matched and subsequently further tailored to be adaptive to a specific user and therapist goal. Custom setup designs include sensor-based input control devices that are worn (e.g., biofeedback), non-invasive (e.g., invisible such as cameras, infrared or ultrasound), or free-standing/or held (e.g., video game controllers). These devices offer various opportunities for alternative means of interaction of various interactive content such as abstract artistic expressions (e.g., painting or music making), robotic devices, or digital video games. More recently, affordable commercial systems such as Sony's Playstation EyeToy®, GestureTek's Interactive Virtual Reality Exercise System (IREX®™) and Nintendo's Wii®™, and others are also used.

The author's created conglomerate system that is in focus in this chapter suggests advancement beyond such commercial game systems for use in healthcare and rehabilitation. The possibility of personalization, i.e. of both feedforward and feedback interaction is directly associated to the decision-making topic of this chapter as this is a need for future efficient systems to optimally motivate participation.

2.1 Adaptive to Individual Needs and Preferences

The concept involves system adaptation according to each user's needs and preferences. Programming flexibility of the created environment/situation (referred to as Virtual Interactive Space (VIS) [7]) enables sensitivity of sourcing human data (mostly motion) to be tailored to the individual and then mapped to responsive medium(s). This is presented in such a way to stimulate the user to react according to a therapeutic training goal. As presented earlier in the chapter, user *afferent-efferent neural feedback loop closure* is suggested achieved in this way (figure 2).

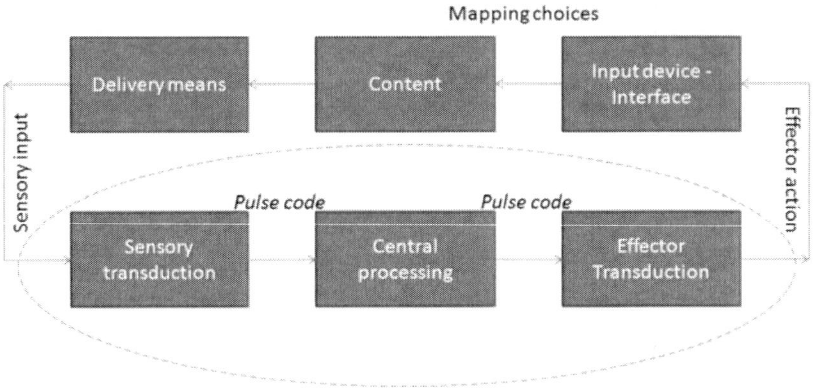

Fig. 2. Afferent-efferent neural feedback loop closure [see also 11]

In figure 2 the dotted oval represents the human and the objects are the data signal processing (DSP). Effectors action is captured by the sensing device and sensory input is presented via display (visuals) or speakers (auditory). Re-programming (configuration change) of the VIS input device and content is according to user reaction and is carried out by the facilitator in the action phase of the session. It is also reflected upon post-session and the system is refined accordingly. By affecting incremental VIS changes, *reafferentation* training is evoked (figure 3). This is a strategy of change where a familiar goal e.g. a sound according to a specific location in space is changed to induce user detection of error, search to correct, and subsequent correction and re-learning of new location. This technique is used to extend movement without engaging at a conscious level. Decisions innate to SoundScapes are evident of facilitator reafferentation strategies for each user and this is optimized through the use of invisible interface technologies [e. g., 7-11]. In other words, this form of training is where familiarity of the location of action effect (i.e. revisited causal - data/feedback -hotspot) is manipulated through facilitator change of system parameter (e.g., head direction/location, sensitivity of sensor). Locations of no-action 'stillness' zones are also designed for PMLD participant communicated "pause", "change", or "end"...etc.

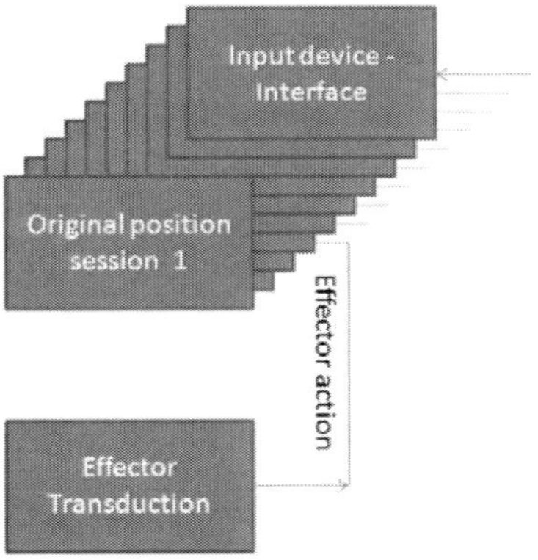

Fig. 3. Reafferentation training: incremental movement change of feedback stimuli

2.2 Facilitator Role: Intervention

A main role of the facilitator in this applied research is to support the user's perception of what can be done. Empowerment of 'doing' is essential for user-experience. As stated previously, in most instances an input device that is based upon technology that is invisible to the human eye is used (e.g., infrared, ultrasound, or camera – figure 1). In these cases the feedback content acts as the direct communicator of feed-forward action and thus becomes the 'perceived interface'. This direct and immediate causal feedback loop, if optimally configured to be interesting and engaging, motivates user participation. However, such engaged motivation can become problematic as user-drift from the interface sensing area can occur, e.g. via over-enthusiasm.

The facilitator must ensure positioning of the means to source the human gesture is optimal (input device location, direction, and setup) along with appropriate content with affordances to guide the user to remain connected to the sensing input device so that perceived 'doing' (i.e. interaction with the multimedia) is intuitive. This also assists motor control training and associated cognitive relations to same. Goal-directed user behavior is targeted via facilitator system-change decisions based upon expert input (therapist, professional healthcare, and/or family/friends) such that user sense of self-agency is achieved that leads to a user sense of empowerment. This inner empowerment is represented externally through non-verbal indicators such as facial responses, eye contact, and interactions. The feedback-feedforward link is thus responsible for ensuring action possibilities available in the environment are evoked as natural. However, even if the VIS is optimally set up as outlined so that the user is immersed in the experience it is meaningless unless the user can perceive what he/she can achieve through participation. This instructive, often demonstrative, facet of facilitator intervention is often overlooked as such instances involve improvisation that often involves physical guidance of the known user abilities alongside knowledge of both the input device (interface) and the mapped content. In-action decision-making is where a system-change is deemed required to maintain and optimize motivation of a user when undergoing a training session with the responsive virtual reality/multimedia system.

On-action decision-making reflects on archived video footage and other triangulated material from a session along with facilitator notes and recall. In-action decision-making is at the sole discretion of the facilitator conducting the session with the participant as these are usually one-to-one[1] with a target to promote self-driven play, i.e. without facilitator intervention. On-action decision-making can involve additional input such as therapist, healthcare professional or even family who can suggest preferences when the user has no verbal ability. The role of facilitator involves intuitive reflection and action in the form of system change based upon close observation of the user's exhibited reactions and emotions, i.e. feedforward, as well as the system response to user input, i.e. feedback. The facilitator role involves using one's own embedded 'enactive knowledge', which associates to tacit knowledge and is 'learned by doing'. It is based on experiences of perceptual responses to action, both from the feedforward (observed user) and feedback (observed system response) perspective. Facilitator action (ongoing decision-making activity) is thus a response to evaluation of user activity that is reactive to the system (and system-change, which is the decision made by the facilitator). In this way Varela's model of 'enactive cognition' [58] is associated. This type of evaluation has been suggested as 'the most direct, in the sense that it is natural and intuitive, since it is based on the experience and on the perceptual responses to motor acts' [25, p. 2].

Decision to change is developed through applying the system in various contexts and then subjecting the decisions and the reasons behind the decision-change to subsequent analysis. Complexities are inherent to such decisions that are based mostly upon subjective evaluation of exhibited user reactions to improvised (experience-guided) intervention. Experiences thus assist such complexities due to learning from making wrong decisions of change system parameters.

2.3 Motivation

Motivation is defined as a feeling of a need to do something [35] and it is this feeling and need that is a goal of design, intervention and refinement in respect of both participant and facilitator in SoundScapes. Included in system use exploration is a dynamic relationship between the inter-related human attributes of 'emotion', 'motivation', and 'movement' (both adapted and non-adapted). Association is through the word emotion deriving from Latin *e movere*, meaning 'to move' or to produce movement. Relationship between emotionality and adapted/non-adapted movement is well-documented in the literature e.g. [35]. Optimization system use is through matching change parameters to an individual profile so that fun is had. Fun relates to joy, which can lead to development [30]. However, emotion, motivation, and movement are all dependent on effective and competent parameter change that does not interrupt participant or facilitator engagement in a session.

[1] Usually the participant's care-person attends the sessions to ensure well-being.

Intrinsic motivation is where engaged participation in a personally challenging activity is just for the sake of participating. This stimulates interest, curiosity, satisfaction and enjoyment without thought of reward [56]. Intrinsic motivation links to the gameplay approach of SoundScapes intervention; it is linked to *autotelic* [55] and *flow* state [15, 16, and 17]. Intrinsic motivation is considered conducive to creative expression, whereas, extrinsic motivation, i.e. reward based, is considered detrimental [2, 3]. Both can be implemented in design/refinement of a SoundScapes session. When extrinsic motivation is required, for example, a created digital painting from gesture-control can be shown to others acting as a simple reward goal [8].

Experiences from sessions suggest that the motivation continuum between intrinsic and extrinsic can be improvised in the intervention phase according to participant profile and responses. However, when the feedback content is optimal and the participant is in flow state, more often than not, the facilitator role is passive. Participant departure from flow promotes increased activity by the facilitator to address participant motivation through parameter change or guidance and support.

Facilitator diligence of participant motivation signifiers is important. Such signifiers are important because they guide the facilitator in his/her intervention strategy.

SoundScapes intervention strategy has evolved through experiential analysis of sessions that have a goal of enriching a life. The strategy is informed through reflective analysis both in-action and on-action, especially of original video recordings, of own experiences, especially mistakes. The next section closes the evaluation section by presenting the model for intervention that has abductively evolved.

2.4 Intervention Model for Decision-Making

A session facilitator is acknowledged as having a key role in intervention with disabled individuals, e.g. [23, pp. 72-74] [40, pp. 49-50]. Improvised intervention, passive or active, is via available system tools (system change parameters made available by session design/refinement). Optimizing participant 'mirroring' is via these resources. Implementing these resources is the foundation of the concept of 'Zone of Optimized Motivation' (ZOOM) (Figure 4).

ZOOM reflects facilitator intervention specific to system use where motivation is optimized (shaded diagonal) and flow state present. It is considered needed to contextualize how knowing the right time for introducing change (δ) can lead to further development [14]. Participant competence over challenge for a period of time can start to wane motivation as familiarity or boredom emerge, recognizing this, the facilitator can change a system parameter so that a new challenge provokes augmented participant input. Changes are participant dependent and flexible along a motivational continuum. In other words, they can be organized around tasks - motivationally extrinsic and discrete, i.e. in steps, or configured to be more intrinsic to motivation perceived as continuous, aimless and exploratory where, seemingly, tasks are self-determined [27]. Incrementing challenge can also provoke motivation/learning collapse in line with Yan and Fischer [62]. When a collapse is recognized, often signified by participant disengagement followed by

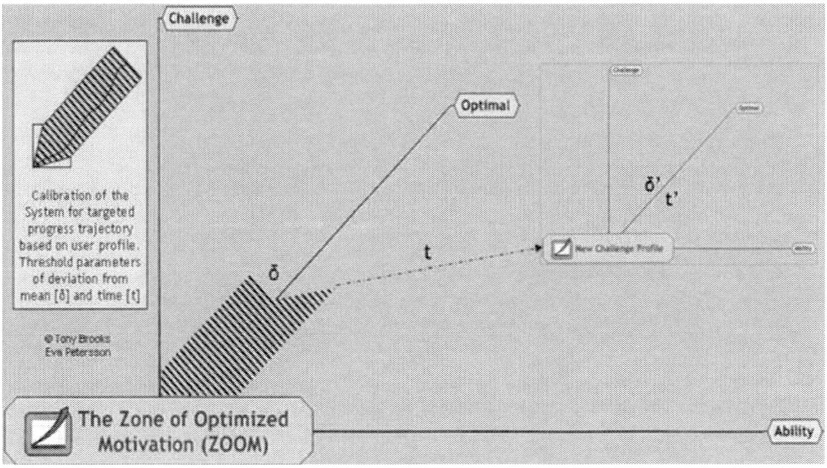

Fig. 4. The Zone of Optimized Motivation (ZOOM)

communicative gesture, the facilitator has to decide on the intervention step of either allowing time (t) for new 'learning' to evolve, or alternatively, to return to a prior challenge level, or even to a preceding (easier) level to again motivate participation. Facilitator experience and knowledge of participant profile guides such decisions. Attending caregiver assists by close observation with the aim of preventing participant over exertion and ensuring well-being.

An experienced participant can also communicate when a change is required, either within the current genre (e.g., sound patch change) or more diverse across modalities (e.g., from music to painting or game). Such a communication is where the participant uses what is referred to as the stillness zone, or non-active area. Such use is an indication of learning in profoundly disabled individuals. The process of facilitating is improvised, iterative and not as clear-cut as may be believed due to participant idiosyncratic traits. Many need initial guidance [49, 50] (physical or imitation) to articulate, especially the inexperienced. Such scaffolding [61] is inherent in the facilitator intervention role.

3 Therapeutic Applications

Rizzolatti and Arbib [48] inform how the human performance system has the capability to observe and recognize motor actions of another individual through neural representations that use the resultant information to map and execute similar actions as imitation. Motor neuron behavior is thus reactive to meaningful visual input. They further inform that the motor system 'resonates' during the observation and they link resonance behavior to *release phenomena, learning and instinct* [57] as well as to 'response facilitation' and cognitive processing [12].

These issues are discussed elsewhere in SoundScapes research and for the sake of brevity are not expanded herein.

In SoundScapes, rather than considering observation and recognition of another individual, a belief is that brain-generated actions are stimulated from recognition (not necessarily consciously recognized) of associations between self-generated feedbacks to feedforward actions that are self-emitted (consciously intended or a subconsciously responsive action to stimulus i.e. not consciously reacted upon but stimulus-driven). Feedback is primary, i.e. self-recognition of feedforward motion, and secondary via the mediating content stimuli that results from the motion. As both feedforward excitation and feedback association are adaptive a form of digital mirroring ensues. This induces closure of the afferent-efferent neural feedback loop [11]. The adaptation of the system-change parameters by the facilitator addresses intention, instinct and reaction interpreted of user input action and reaction. The reaction informs of user motivation, interest and engagement and it is these cumulated representations that act as guide to facilitator improvised control of the system.

A metaphor to this facilitator role is of a puppeteer who manipulates the strings to control interactions, in this case the available system parameters are as the puppeteer strings and the puppet is the user. However, the metaphor is temporary as the user reacts to perceived system affordances and develops recognition of causal competence that result in sense of self-agency, which leads to inner-empowerment that becomes externally represented. A form of micro-development ensues that relates to learning according to system design and therapist goal. However, system-change parameters are under the control of the facilitator and often mistakes are made of when to change and to what extent the increment of change should be. Over the years this has been a learnt process that is ongoing. Reflective of this acknowledgement is the emergent model titled Zone of Optimized Motivation (ZOOM).

3.1 Evaluation

Evaluating system use includes assessing participant response, and this is acknowledged as complex [33]. In line with [37, 38] qualitative inductive research methodologies were researched and selected to be integrated with the goal to create a flexible, multidimensional model to critically understand what was involved in system use. Background and development of the emergent model for intervention and evaluation is presented in the following sections.

SoundScapes has been evaluated to enhance social interactions, competence development, and cognitive/physical improvements [7, 39]. Participant awareness of enhancement, along with fun from interactions, both with system and facilitator, contribute to motivation. Change is targeted through intervention and is acknowledged in Action Research methodology. The next section introduces Action Research as an element of the method foundation.

3.2 Action Research

Figure 5 illustrates two sequential iterations of an Action Research process. Kemmis & McTaggart [31] describe Action Research as a "spiral of self-reflective cycles of planning a change, acting and observing the process and consequences of the change, reflecting on these processes and consequences, and then re-planning, acting and observing, reflecting, and so on…" (p. 595). In SoundScapes it is considered a social model e.g., due to how planning considers influence of attendees, that fits well with the activity theory framework described earlier. In this research it contributes as a sequential 'interactive inquiry process' [44]. Environments are both the physical situations where sessions take place and the virtual environments that are encountered in the session. Facilitator attention is acknowledged as influential in case studies conducted under an action research methodology that involves action and learning [36]. Curry [18] informs how "action research requires trust, openness, high tolerance for uncertainty and surprise" (p. 6). These have been found as key aspects in this specific intervention with disabled people.

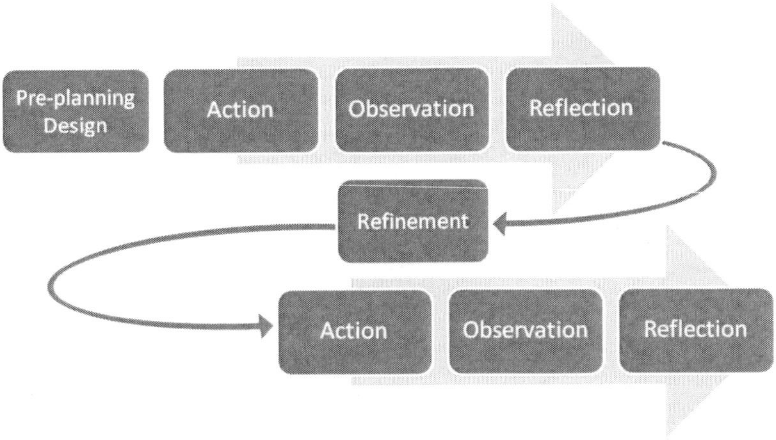

Fig. 5. Example of two iterations of Action Research process

To satisfy the investigation the temporal linear/sequential profile of Action Research required enriching thus a synthesis with a second approach having an opposing non-linear recursive profile was made. Mahoney [35] relates how motivation theorists suggest hypothetical tensions resulting in polarized concepts or operations promote activity and learning. The multidimensional profile that has evolved is illustrated in figures 6(a-p) on pages 156-161. Evaluation was recursive considering both linear and non-linear dimensions of archived triangulated material, which assisted both in-action and on-action reflective analysis [53, 54]. Hermeneutic enquiry was found fitting to complement Action Research, especially as the approach could be interpreted to investigate systemically between part and whole to explore dynamic relationships [21].

3.3 Hermeneutic Spiral

Hermeneutics is a flexible core interpretive tool suitable for retrospective reflection of whole and part [28, p. 134], and is acknowledged as an iterative strategy creating knowledge and knowing [1]. The focus is upon the relationship between the whole and the parts, which are dependent on each other, and together they create understanding. The approach was considered complementary to Action Research and the iterative research and development profile of SoundScapes. Schleirmacher [52] had an emphasis on knowledge creation through the hermeneutic circle as a dialectic movement between part and whole with an emphasis on understanding in relation to modes of communication. In other words, understanding of the whole by reference to the individual parts and understanding each individual part by reference to the whole. His focus was on how the interpreter was important in the process of interpretation and for successful interpretation prior understanding was involved. [26] also emphasized that a necessity was pre-understanding within the process of understanding and accordingly extended the hermeneutic circle as a spiral; thus with a temporal form. The act of interpretation, i.e. the giving of meaning to something, has a time dimension and thus, in SoundScapes, interpretation of data is via forward sequential Action Research complemented by the retrospectively non-linear hermeneutic approach. Interpretation is of activity, user-experience, and learning.

The importance placed on reflection of how experiences between an individual and an environment can support development is not new [5, 32]. The synthesis of method (action research) and approach (hermeneutics) conducted as 'recursive reflection' is in line with Eden and Huxham [22, p. 81] who state how it is crucial that an appropriate degree of reflection is built into process, and that the process includes a means of holding on to that reflection. Further, Brooker et al. [6] attempted enriching outcomes of action research through a Hermeneutic spiral in a different context.

3.4 Hermeneutic Action Research Recursive Reflection

Resulting inductively from explorative enquiry to influence and support decision-making in virtual healthcare and rehabilitation is an emergent evaluation model titled 'Hermeneutic Action Research Recursive Reflection'. The term 'Recursive' is used fitting the iterative model of enquiry where all original material is available to be analyzed and continuously reanalyzed in light of new knowledge gain. 'Reflection' is used in reference to how experiences evolve into learning. The model involves the creation of an (all data) archive, i.e. a repository consisting of session notes, participant journals, video recordings, interviews, questionnaires, concept/mind maps, in other words all triangulated materials resulting from sessions. Subsequent evaluations and re-evaluations add to the archive. The process of Recursive Reflection is central to Hermeneutic Action Research as it signifies process of reflective analysis. The following figure sequence (denoted as figure 6a-p) illustrates how the Recursive Reflection model is flexible to address session-to-session analysis and refinement.

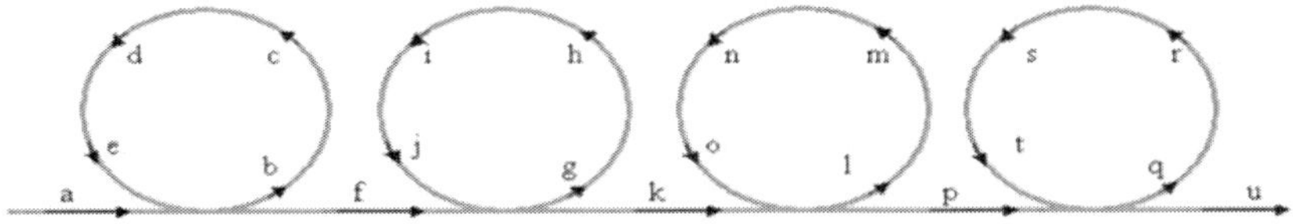

Fig. 6(a). Illustrates a typical four cycle/session action research profile. This consists of sequential segments:- (1) planning a change via action [segment a]; (2) action – the actual session with participant [segment a-to-b]; (3) post-session observation of the action [b-c]; (4) reflection on the action [c-d]; (5) refining – e.g. of the created system set-up or strategies to address the natural systems [d-e], and (6) the planning for the next action [e-f]… and so on for the other cycles.

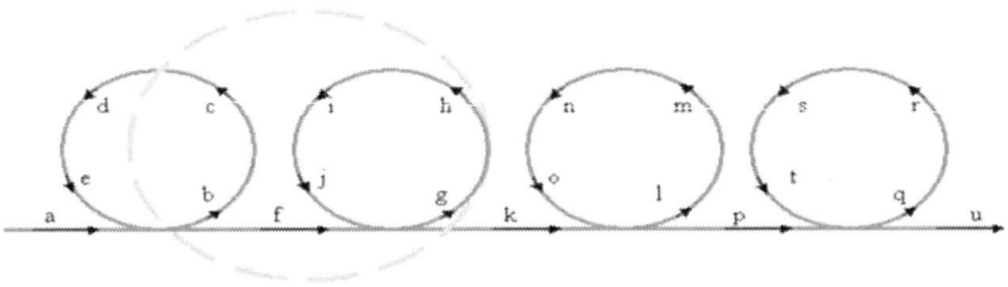

Fig. 6(b). This is the same four-cycle Action Research sequence plus a single retrospective hermeneutic on-action recursive reflection (shown as dotted line of anticlockwise direction). Initiated from a point in time during the observation segment [g-h] on action [f-g]; this indicates that prior session recall [a-e] was stimulated with most recent data acquisition [f-g] to prompt a researcher decision to initiate a secondary reflection on the initial session archive. In other words, what was learnt from experiencing action [f-g] stimulated a recursive reflection of preceding session action and observation. This process is illustrated in the figure by the start of the dotted line emitting upward and anticlockwise from the observation segment [g-h]. Retrospective reflection of the prior session includes the researcher consulting previous session notes, videos and other triangulated material. This reflection is 'on-action' segment [a-b]. The researcher then has additional material informing to the research as a whole, as well as to the second action cycle/session [f-j]. Findings augment observation segment [g-h] of session action [f-g], subsequently improving the reflections in segment [h-i], and ultimately influencing refinement in [i-j] and next iteration planning [j-k]...etc.

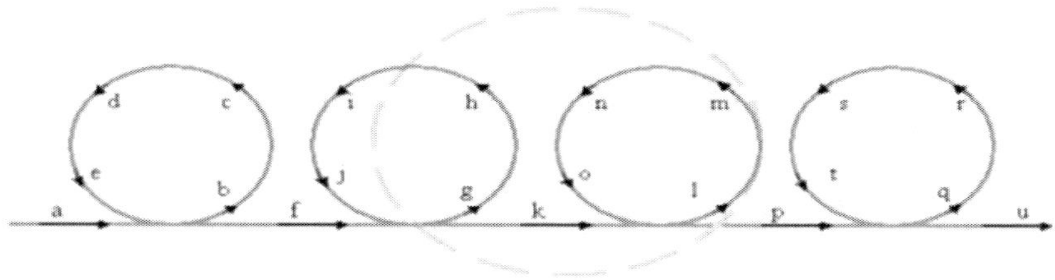

Fig 6(c). Four-cycle Action Research sequence integrated with a single hermeneutic 'on-action recursive reflection' (shown as dotted line of anticlockwise direction). This reflection initiates from a point in time located between [l-m] but instead originating from the third session observation segment as a reflection on the second session action segment [f-g].

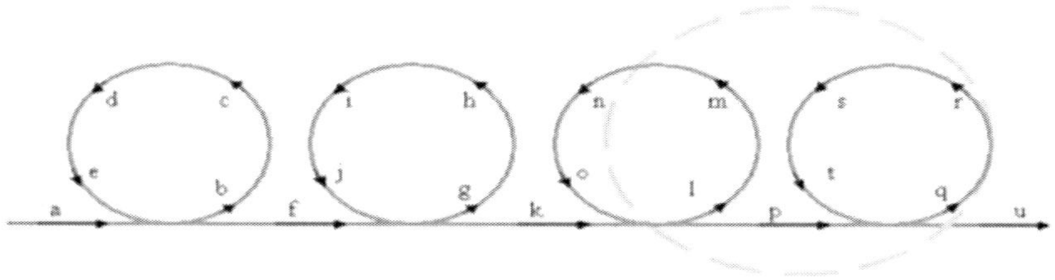

Fig. 6(d). Similar to above but initiated from the fourth session observation segment [q-r] in respect of 'on-action recursive reflection' of the third session action segment [k-l]

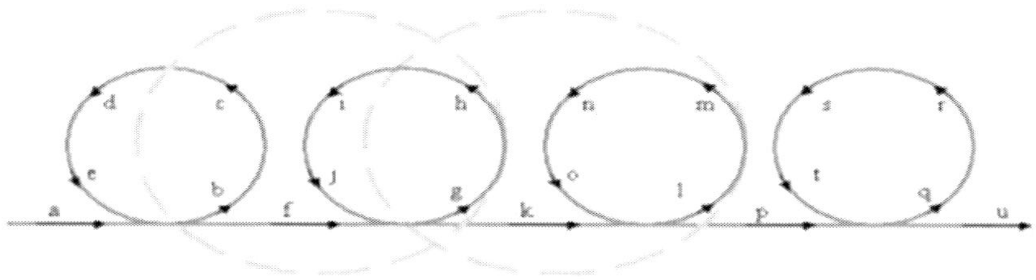

Fig. 6(e). Two iterations of the retrospective hermeneutic 'on-action recursive reflection' are shown where additional knowledge was believed available from the first session [a-e] based upon what had been observed in the second session [f-j]. Similarly, the second session offered additional learning for the third session.

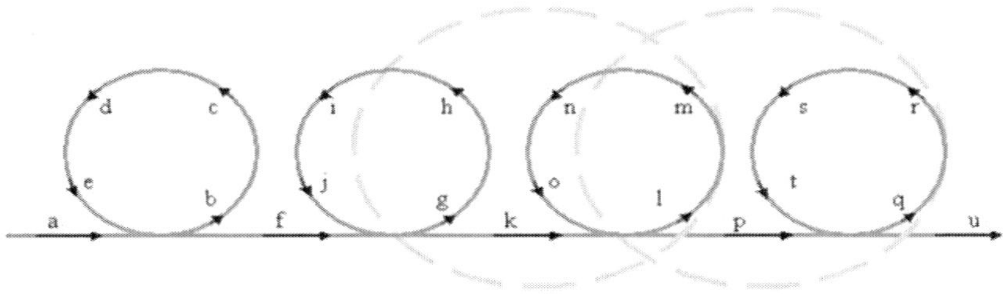

Fig. 6(f). Two iterations of the retrospective hermeneutic 'on-action recursive reflection' are shown originating from session 3 and session 4 observation segments respectively

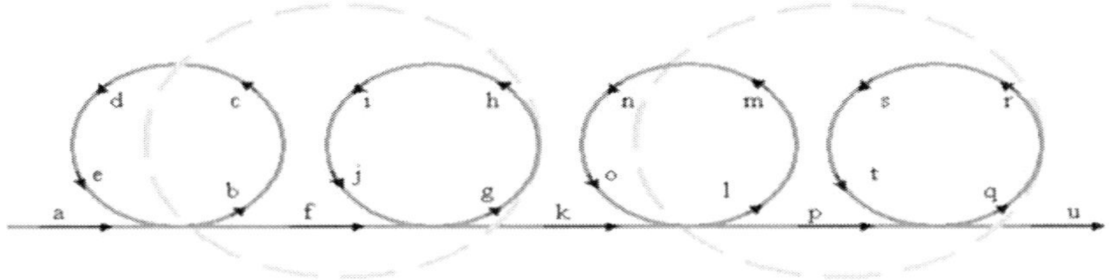

Fig. 6(g). Two iterations of the retrospective hermeneutic 'on-action recursive reflection' are shown originating from session 2 and session 4 observation segments respectively

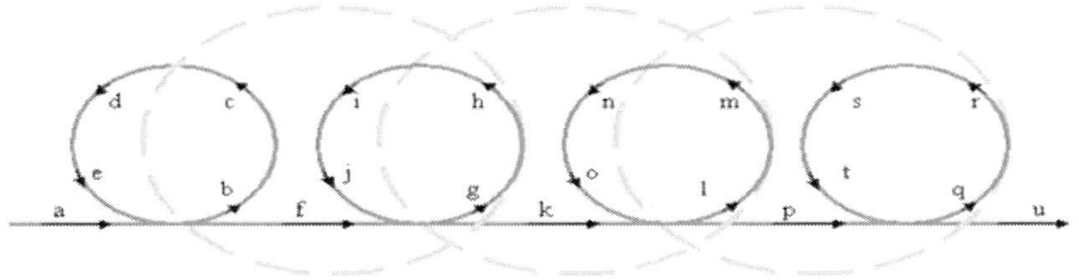

Fig. 6(h). Triple hermeneutic 'on-action recursive reflection' over a four session program where each subsequent session is systematically accesses prior session data

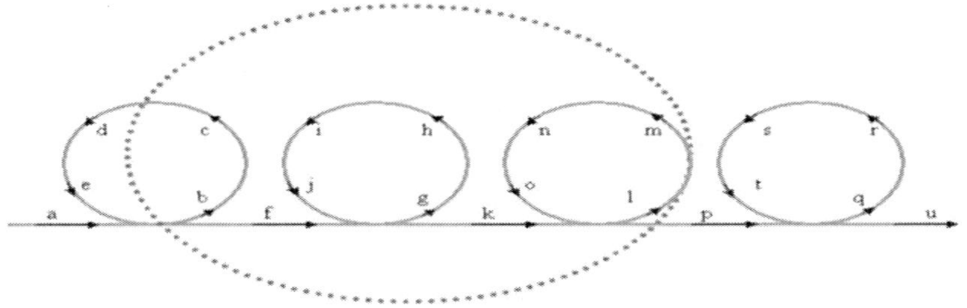

Fig. 6(i, j, k). Above and the next two images illustrate further examples of single and double retrospective hermeneutic 'on-action recursive reflection' applied upon an action research four session program. These illustrate that the model is not limited to retrospective sequential application as application is from any session in respect of any prior session.

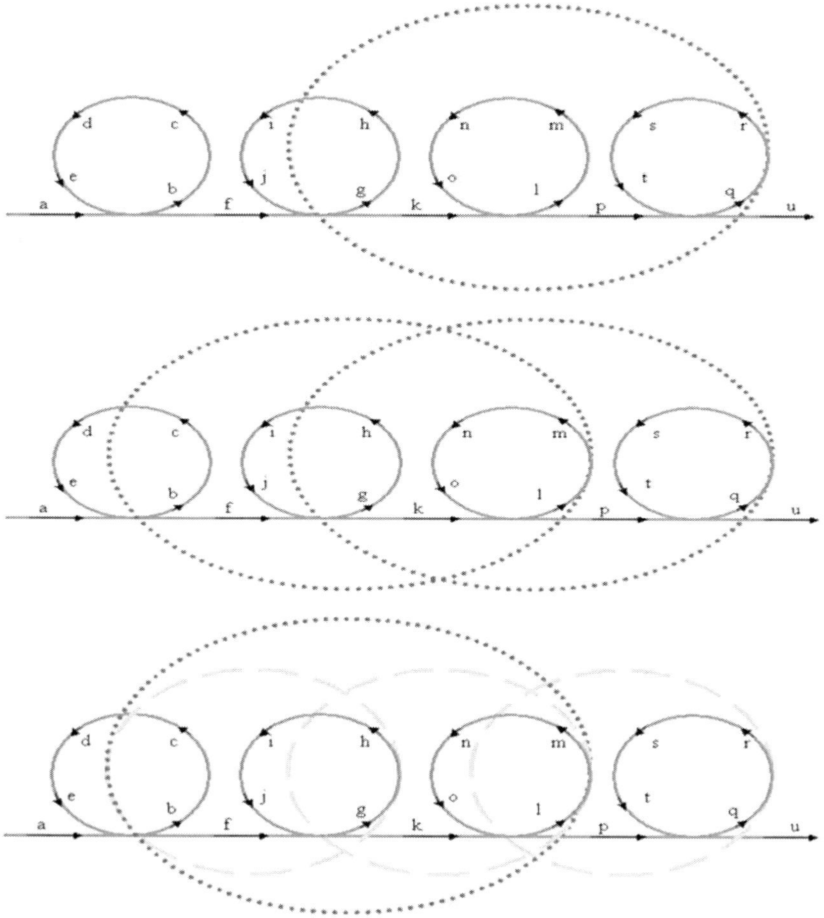

Fig. 6(l). Preceding figures illustrate retrospective 'single non-sequential' combined with a 'triple sequential' hermeneutic 'on-action recursive reflection' applied over a four-session action research sequence. The above figure interpretation reads as either:-

(1) Initial findings from the observation phase [l-m] of the third session action promoted an additional 'on-action recursive reflection' upon the first session, which was then brought into the observation segment of the third session, which in turn promoted an 'on-action recursive reflection' upon the second session action,

– [a-b-c-d-e-f-g-ω-h-i-j-k-l-ω-m-n-o-ω'-p-q-ω-r-s-t-u] ...or

(2) Findings following the reflection and refinement on the third session promoted an additional 'on-action recursive reflection' upon the first session before a satisfactory planning for the fourth section was completed -

[a-b-c-d-e-f-g-ω-h-i-j-k-l-ω'-m-n-o-ω-p-q-ω-r-s-t-u]

…where omega [ω] represents a retrospective sequential hermeneutic ‘on-action recursive reflection’ and omega’ [ω’] represents a ‘single non-sequential’ hermeneutic ‘on-action recursive reflection’. Thus the model is flexible in that the hermeneutic ‘on-action recursive reflection’ can be following the session action of after a full review of the session.

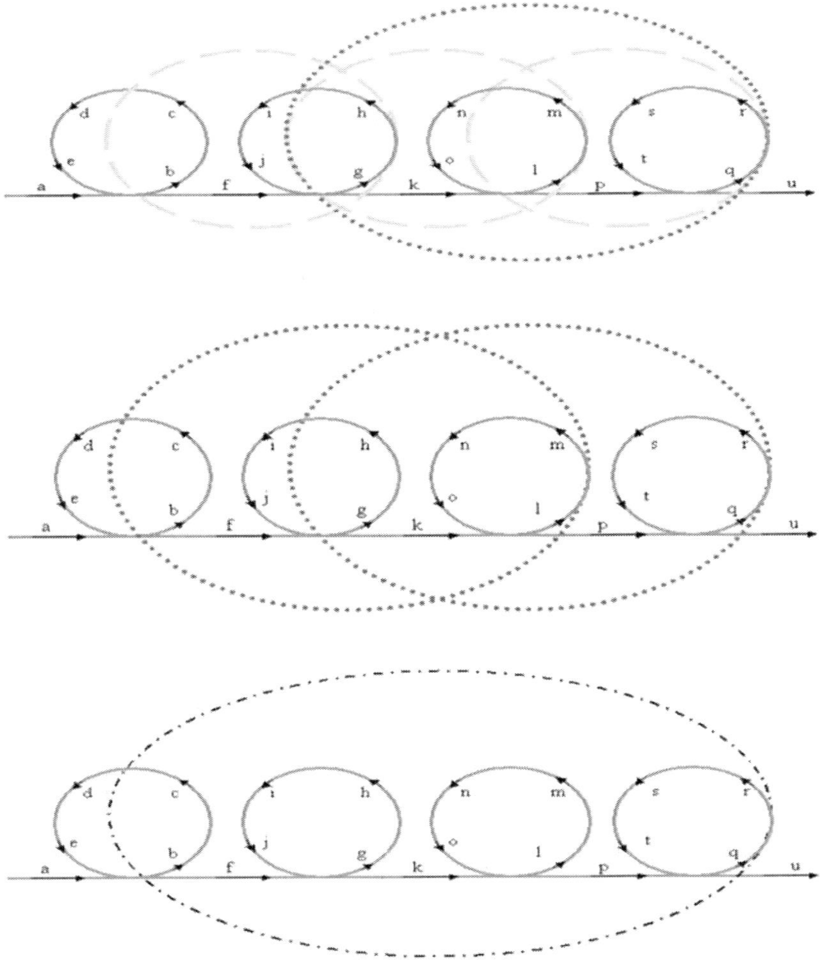

Fig. 6(m, n, o). These figures above illustrate examples of non-sequential’ hermeneutic ‘on-action recursive reflection’. An emergent model for systematic evaluation of subjective data has evolved out of an attempt to elicit maximum session data to inductively inform and evolve the research theories – see final (next) image with all options illustrated.

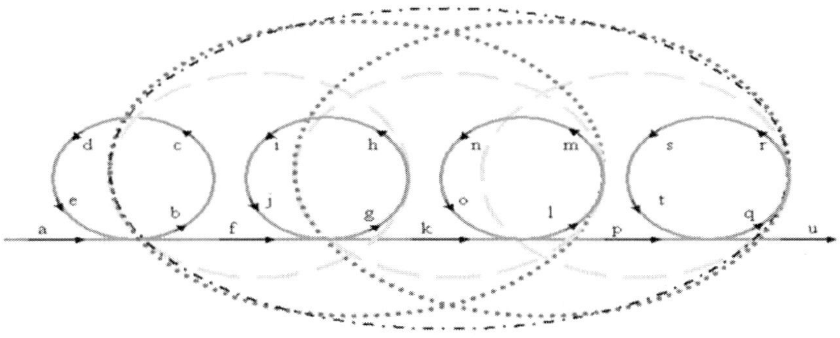

Fig. 6(p). Illustrates multidimensional flexibility of the concept to enable eliciting of maximum understanding from original material - indicated by multiplicity of theoretically available recursive channels (various dotted line ovals radiating from observation phases). This model informs and supports decisions on design and refinement.

3.5 Informed Design and Refinement

Participant action relative to system feedback is a common unit of analysis in SoundScapes. A session facilitator conducts both 'in-action' and 'on-action' assessment - the latter usually with the participant's therapist. Assessment is informed by e.g., facial expressions, non-verbal body language, and utterances. Additional assessment is available though involving 'significant others', e.g., healthcare professional, teacher, therapist or family/friend. As these people know the participants outside of a test situation i.e. Activities of Daily Living (ADLs), their insights assist in assessments, which leads to evaluations that inform the system design refinement for next sessions with each specific participant.

Design and refinement includes making decisions on what is included as available for a facilitator to change in-action. System change parameters affect dynamic relationships as well as system whole and parts. Too many change parameters can lead to redundancy while insufficient reduces flexibility and potential for participant development that may arise. An example of this is when numerous banks of auditory sound patches are used as feedback content making selection overly arduous and operation inefficient.

This chapter informs of an original concept and the motion-sensitive interactive system created as an open research vehicle. Research investigated a supplementary tool for therapists to motivate and enhance disabled users' participation in training. Empowering disabled people to control (physical or digital) artifacts was envisioned to motivate training of whatever body processes were involved in that control thereby offering a non-traditional tool to augment control of that competence. Afferent-efferent neural loop closure and reafferentation training are presented. Apparatus and method have developed along parallel lines through explorative enquiry.

As an open-ended system that is configurable across sensing, mapping, and stimuli, system parameter change variables enable mixing and matching to an individual's profile or therapist goal. Novel non-invasive sensor-based prototypes were created specific for the research and original algorithms were made to facilitate optimal mapping to multimedia content that include audiovisual and robotic device as stimuli.

Overall, response to the work has been positive and related work corroborate potentials through report of participant increased joint-activities, augmented social interaction, and acquiring progressive capacities including 'self-recognized achievement' and 'enhanced sense of control' [e.g., 34, p. 33]. However, system operation/change is problematic for staff, especially when configured beyond a basic system. Reports from use of the 'SoundScapes Room' commissioned in 1999 with staff training and evaluation of use included are of continued use. However, even this basic system a decade later is problematic. If they are not familiar with technology and do not get allocated time to learn it will remain problematic. Thus the models presented in this chapter point to how decisions are made and tentatively suggest how machine supported intervention can assist staff in operation and optimization of practices.

Having a manifold role as inventor/designer/facilitator/researcher included reconfiguring system parameters in the sessions with a significant other (caregiver, therapist, family member, and/or teacher) in attendance. However, training significant others to operate has been problematic as many caregivers proved to be technophobic, unfamiliar or simply not interested in technology – despite the observed positive outcomes. Technical apparatus setup – system apparatus and multiple camera analysis (MCA) system [11], operation and reconfiguration (especially in-action); and the systematic archiving of data for post-session annotation and evaluation were all found problematic for staff who generally were untrained in use of such technology. The emergent model for intervention and evaluation is offered as a first step towards supporting new training that is envisaged required in the field to support optimal use of such technical tools. Therapist training and applied collaborations with digital artist/programmers are foreseen as a direction for next generation practitioners.

3.6 Commercial Products

Commercially available and affordable sensor-based game controllers have recently been adopted into physical training and rehabilitation. Around 2003 the Sony EyeToy was introduced as a single motion-sensing technology device (optical) that enabled control of video game artifacts.

A limited number of studies explored using this device but a common restriction was inaccessible motion data and game content e.g. [9, 43]. Subsequently, Nintendo introduced the Wii platform and game controllers, especially the "Wiimote" and "WiiFit balance board". These are increasingly being adopted in rehabilitation training [24, 29] and education where motivation is reported [4].

Importantly, the controllers allow access to motion data making it available for mapping to control independent content and to archive for analysis to support decision-making. This data stream is also then available to also input to machine-learning of interaction.

3.7 Corroborated Outcomes

Ellis (1995-2004) presents observations of participation progression included from involuntary to voluntary, from accidental to intended, from indifference to interest, from confined to expressive, from random to purposeful, from gross to fine, from exploratory to preconceived, from isolated to integrated, from solitary to individual Whilst terminologies are entities that remain open for subjective interpretation I suggest close corroboration between our findings. The findings point to commonalities of user-experiences, responses, and participant progression that are not limited to specific feedback content or specific input device profile. Simple 'fun doings' experienced as 'magic' emerging from a designed situation matched to a personal profile would seem a key aspect. Important is that the technology needs to be indiscernible and capable of enabling a transparent experience of control of directly and immediately responsive pleasurable content. This then acts as the interface to achieve the desired experience. Decision-making of how to design, refine, and - in sessions - fine-tune the user experience opportunities are key to the work and emanate from facilitator experiences. Machine-supported decision-making to support related investigation and practices is a challenge that lays ahead as such support will assist the burden predicted of future societal demographic dynamics.

In traditional rehabilitation training intervention is focused upon targeting specific impaired skills believed as being the root of dysfunction. Facilitator-led sessions conducted under an *interventionist-centered approach* target achievement of discrete goals and outcomes without consideration of the idiosyncratic preferences, desires, likes and dislikes of the user e.g. [51]. In the author's research, a *whole person approach* is implemented so that the facilitator is responsive to user needs and desires where decisions of system-change targets user-experiences of interaction in activities that are meaningful, interesting and pleasurable. These needs can be user-communicated in-action or resultant from on-action analysis. Under this premise individuals are more likely to be curious, engaged, and activated to participate through articulating via their residual abilities/assets [19]. Thus, design is of situations, interactions and interventions that can support optimizing user motivated participation toward making sense of cause (human feedforward input and subsequent reaction) and effect (content feedback response). Optimized user motivation thus relates to system design where activity challenge is balanced to user skill level, which subsequently relates to aesthetic resonance. Exhibited aesthetic resonance represents achieving closure of the afferent-efferent neural feedback loop towards developing existing assets or acquiring new skills. In this way opportunities to augment a users' understanding about own abilities where their sense of mastery is improved become apparent [41]. Motivated participation can also be a result of user enjoyment from appealing qualities of the created situation or context that attract user interest and curiosity to attract involvement [45]. A created VIS environment stimulates immediate responses to gestures that are designed to please to such an extent that participants become unaware of the effort involved in the generation of movement. Motivation to move resulting from pleasurable and meaningful experiences stimulates motor activities that can have communicational value via associated gestures and expressed representations that often go unnoticed yet in this research they are subject of recursive reflection of exhibited aesthetic resonance. This chapter questions what may be needed in order for a machine to analyze the created situation to support the facilitator and team in making automatic decisions of system-change to assist. The challenge lies in the ability of the machine to interpret innate complexities of subjective evaluation of human behavior and to act upon these interpretations so as to learn idiosyncratic characteristics of the user to effect decisions of system-change.

4 Machine-Supported Intervention

Virtual Reality suggests benefits of use including that it is safe and does not tire or get bored with repetitive mundane activities that may otherwise influence motivation of both user and facilitator [20, 42, 43, 46, and 59]. Contemporary interactive virtual environments are increasingly used in healthcare and rehabilitation. For example, video games[2] are more prevalent in the field following their recent use of untraditional input devices that escape confines of mouse, joystick, and keyboard. Unlike earlier examples, contemporary video games have instructions embedded into the game start (as opposed to manuals that should be read) that enable players to quickly understand input device cause and effect. Often a dedicated opening sequence takes the player through calibration and control of the input device followed by the gameplay situation via examples and demos that are often followed by an initial training challenge. Gameplay then progresses such that as a user achieves a level a subsequent level is presented that offers increased challenges so that skill is augmented. However, many games are limited in their flexibility to address individual users, especially those with special needs/disability. Input devices are programmed to specific interactions with specific content and incremental level challenge may not reflect nuance of skill progression which relates to microdevelopment [62]. Software such as GlovePIE (PC & Linux)[3] or OSCulator (Mac)[4] can improve the situation by enabling parameter mapping of an input device such as the commonly used Wiimote. However, the interaction is still limited to mapping options that can be accessed for content control and such mappings have to be meaningful for the session/program therapeutic goals. Such 'hacking' is often beyond the competences and desires of healthcare professionals and weaknesses in robustness of such ad-hoc setups tends to also limit the appeal for practitioners to explore such solutions that could address flexibility to individual needs. The open system that has been used as the core in the author's research utilizes three robust technologies to capture gesture in an unencumbered untraditional way. Camera, Ultrasound and Infrared technologies are used to designate invisible active zones to source human motion data from gesture. Each has a distinct profile of capture that can be programmed to each individual's need. The profiles are planar, linear and volumetric and each technique of use offers plusses and minuses in use as an input device to control multimedia content. Applied in the field of rehabilitation non-intuitive technologies have been found to motivate participation

[2] e.g., http://www.usatoday.com/tech/science/2008-02-08-wii-rehabilitation_N.htm

[3] http://carl.kenner.googlepages.com/glovepie

[4] http://www.osculator.net

as they can be programmed to address weaknesses in dexterity and usability is efficient and effective as no additional strength is required to hold or operate an interface. Early investigations prior to contemporary computer vision advances focused on ultrasound and infrared. Both technologies enabled non-computer application so that a facilitator could change system parameters quickly with minimum distraction to the user so as to maintain continuity of contact. Unfortunately it must be said that following extensive observations of use many practitioners are not conversant enough with such interactive systems to be able to evoke fullest potentials for their use which could improve benefits to end-users. Potentials of imitation as a strategy for healthcare and rehabilitation training through interactive virtual reality environments as outlined in this chapter are complex. Relating to the animal kingdom [13] reported how imitation can result in an increase in the frequency of an already acquired motor pattern; can change response orientation in space ('response facilitation'), or even modify the motor pattern of an already acquired action ('action-level imitation'). Whiten [60] reports on how sequential relations between actions can be changed by imitation ('sequence imitation').

Advances in computer vision enable machine recognition of facial expressions and other telling non-verbal bodily reactions to such causal interactions, for example pupil reaction to stimuli, mouth shape, etc. Data streams from user input can be archived to cross-reference to such reactions. Content that affects the user in specific ways can also be synchronized and associated to input data and user reaction. One can imagine how advances in Computer Artificial Intelligence could use such cumulated data and with multi-disciplinary input develop an autonomous support system for assisting in therapeutic situations as outlined in this chapter. A reference intelligent machine systems model with adaptive behavior for real time control change has been proposed[5]. The challenge in this context would seem to be in successfully interpreting all of the data to evoke system parameter change which at the moment is a highly subjective operation due to the complexities of the user interaction and intrinsic and extrinsic variables that can influence session intervention. Such a system, if successful, could enable many more 'next generation' therapists and healthcare givers to introduce interactive technology/multimedia systems into their practice without worry of being alienated of the technology. Strengths & weaknesses exist when making decisions of system devices, protocols and mappings. It is often too much to ask families, carers or even therapists to have needed competences to optimize use of such technology in training and learning. Thus, a specialist training studio is established in Denmark to assist families and to train the trainers. In-session decisions of change that are involved can at the moment only rely on the person leading the session. This can also be the user. Mistakes of parameter-change become evident through experience with the system under this approach to intervention. Automated system decision-making would augment the potentials for such situations. Such progress in the field would support families and self-driven home-training applications. In healthcare, participant activity and motivation are becoming increasingly important as is indicated by the levels of obesity, injuries and disease. In education new

[5] http://www.isd.mel.nist.gov/documents/albus/engineeringmind-96.pdf

paradigms are in place that utilizes the power of interactive digital multimedia into curricula, many involve human performance activities. In both cases, healthcare and education, a tool to supplement by supporting decision-making in an automatic way is seen as advancing state-of-the-art.

References

1. Alvesson, M., Sköldberg, K.: Tolkning och reflection: Vetenskapfilosofi och kvalitativ metod. Studentlitteratur, Swedish, Lund (1994)
2. Amabile, T.M.: The social psychology of creativity. Springer, New York (1983)
3. Amabile, T.M.: Creativity in context: Update to the Social Psychology of Creativity. Westview, Boulder (1996)
4. Bailey, C., Pearson, E.: The Nintendo Wii Games Console and its potential for Supporting Disabled Learners in Education. In: Bastiaens, T., Carliner, S. (eds.) Proc. of World Conference on E-Learning in Corporate, Government, Healthcare, and Higher Education, pp. 213–217 (2007)
5. Boud, D., Keogh, R., Walker, D.: Reflection: Turning Experience Into Learning. Routledge, London (1985)
6. Brooker, R., Macpherson, I., Aspland, T.: Enriching the outcomes of action research: Connecting the local with the global through a hermeneutic spiral. Queensland Journal of Educational Research 17(1), 16–28 (2001)
7. Brooks, A.L.: Virtual interactive space (V.I.S.) as a movement capture interface tool giving multimedia feedback for treatment and analysis. In: Proc. World Confederation for Physical therapy, p. 66 (1999)
8. Brooks, A.L., Hasselblad, S.: Creating aesthetically resonant environments for the handicapped, elderly and rehabilitation: Sweden. In: Proc. 6th International Conference on Disability, Virtual Reality and Associated Technologies, pp. 191–198 (2004)
9. Brooks, A.L., Petersson, E.: Play Therapy Utilizing the Sony EyeToy®. In: Slater, M. (ed.) Annual International Workshop on Presence (8th), Presence2005, pp. 303–314. University College London, London (2005)
10. Brooks, A.L., Sorensen, C.: Communication Method and Apparatus. USPTO Patent Full-Text and Image Database: Patent number US 6,893,407 (2005)
11. Brooks, A.L., Hasselblad, S., Camurri, A., Canagarajah, N.: Interaction with shapes and sounds as a therapy for special needs and rehabilitation. In: Proc. 4th Int. Conference on Disability, Virtual Reality, and Associated Technologies, Veszprém, Hungary, pp. 205–212 (2002)
12. Byrne, R.W.: The Thinking Ape. Evolutionary Origins of Intelligence. Oxford University Press, Oxford (1995)
13. Byrne, R.W., et al.: Learning by imitation: A hierarchical approach. Behavioral and Brain Sciences 21(5), 667–721 (1998)
14. Christensen, A.-L., Uzzell, B.P. (eds.): International Handbook of Neuropsychological Rehabilitation. Springer, New York (1999)
15. Csíkszentmihályi, M.: Creativity: Flow and the Psychology of Discovery and Invention. Harper Collins, New York (1997)
16. Csíkszentmihályi, M.: Flow: The classic work on how to achieve happiness. Random House, London (2002)

17. Csíkszentmihályi, M.: Flow: the Psychology of Optimal Experience. Harper Perennial, New York (1991)
18. Curry, A.: Action Research in Action: Involving Students and Professionals. In: World Library and Information Congress: 71th IFLA General Conference and Council (2005)
19. Dunst, C.J.: An integrated framework for practicing early childhood intervention and family support. Perspectives in Education 22(2), 1–16 (2004)
20. Dvorkin, A.Y., Shahar, M., Weiss, P.L.: Reaching within Video-Capture Virtual Reality: Using Virtual Reality as a Motor Control Paradigm. CyberPsychology and Behavior 9(2), 133–136 (2006)
21. Eaglestone, B., Bamidis, P.D.: Music composition for the multi-disabled: A systems perspective. Disab. Human Develop. 7(1), 19–24 (2008)
22. Eden, C., Huxham, C.: Action research for management research. British Journal of Management 7, 75–86 (1996)
23. Ellis, P.: Moving Sound. In: MacLachlan, M., Gallagher, P. (eds.) Enabling Technologies in Rehabilitation: Body Image and Body Function, Churchill Livingstone, Oxford, pp. 59–75 (2004)
24. Ellis, P., Van Leeuwen, L., Brown, K.: Visual-Music Vibrations Improving quality of life for the elderly and children with special needs. Digital Creativity 19(3), 194–202 (2008)
25. Frisoli, A., Camurri, A.: Multisensory interaction in virtual environments. Virtual Reality 10(1), 2–3 (2006)
26. Gadamer, H.G.: Truth and Method, 2nd edn. Continuum International, London (1989)
27. Gaver, W., Bowers, J., Boucher, A., Gellerson, H., Pennington, S., Schmidt, A., Steed, A., Villar, N., Walker, B.: The Drift Table: Designing for ludic engagement. In: Proc. CHI 2004 Design Expo. ACM Press, New York (2004)
28. Gray, C., Malins, J.: Visualizing Research: A Guide to the Research process in Art and Design. Ashgate, Aldershot (2004)
29. Halton, J.: Virtual rehabilitation with video games: A new frontier for occupational therapy. Occupational Therapy Now 10(1), 12–14 (2008), `http://www.caot.ca/otnow/jan%2008/virtual.pdf`
30. Izard, C.: Human Emotions. Plenum, New York (1977)
31. Kemmis, S., McTaggart, R.: Participatory action Research. In: Denzin, N.K., Lincoln, Y.S. (eds.) The Handbook of Qualitative Research, 2nd edn., pp. 567–606. Sage, London (2000)
32. Kreppner, K.: William L. Stern, 1871–1938: A Neglected Founder of Developmental Psychology. Developmental Psychology 28(4), 539–547 (1992)
33. Lampton, D.R., Bliss, J.P., Morris, C.S.: Human Performance Measurement in Virtual Environments. In: Stanney, K.M. (ed.) Handbook of Virtual Environments: Design, Implementation, and Applications, pp. 701–720. LEA, New Jersey (2002)
34. Lopes-dos-Santos, P., Teixeira, L.M., Silva, M., Azeredo, M., Barbosa, M.: Exploring interpersonal dynamics between adults and motor disabled children within aesthetic resonant environments. In: Cobb, S., Brooks, A.L., Sharkey, P.M., Merrick, J. (eds.) International Journal on Disability and Human Development, vol. 5(2), pp. 133–139 (2006)
35. Mahoney, M.J.: Human change processes. Basic Books, New York (1991)
36. McNiff, J., Whitehead, J.: Action Research: Living Theory. Sage, London (2006)
37. Patton, M.: Qualitative evaluation and research methods. Sage, Thousand Oaks (1990)
38. Patton, M.: Utilization-focused evaluation: The new century text. Sage, Thousand Oaks (1997)

39. Petersson, E.: Non-Formal Learning Through Ludic Engagement within Interactive Environments. [Doctoral Thesis] 'Malmö Studies in Educational Sciences', Malmö högskola, Lärarutbildningen / Lund University, Sweden (2006)
40. Pollini, A.: Experimenting with an Ubiquitous Computing Open Architecture. [Doctoral Thesis, Telematica e Società dell 'Informazione Cicle XX. Uni. of Florence and Uni. of Siena] (2008), http://www.ist-palcom.org/publications/files/PhD-Thesis-Pollini.pdf
41. Raab, M., Dunst, C.J.: Influence of child interests on variations in child behavior and functioning. Bridges 4(4), 1–22 (2006)
42. Rand, D., Kizony, R., Feintuch, U., Katz, N., Josman, N., Rizzo, A., Weiss, P.L.: Comparison of Two VR Platforms for Rehabilitation: Video Capture versus HMD. Presence: Teleoperators & Virtual Environments 14(2), 147–160 (2005)
43. Rand, D., Kizony, R., Weiss, P.L.: Virtual reality rehabilitation for all: Vivid GX versus Sony PlayStation II EyeToy. In: Sharkey, P., McCrindle, R., Brown, D. (eds.) International Conference on Disability, Virtual Reality and Associated Technologies, pp. 87–94. University of Reading, Reading (2004)
44. Reason, P., Bradbury, H. (eds.): Handbook of Action Research. Sage, London (2001)
45. Renninger, K.A.: Individual interest and its implications for understanding intrinsic motivation. In: Sansone, C., Harackiewicz, J.M. (eds.) Intrinsic and Extrinsic Motivation: The Search for Optimal Motivation and Performance, pp. 373–404. Academic Press, San Diego (2000)
46. Rizzo, A., Kim, G.: A SWOT Analysis of the Field of Virtual Reality Rehabilitation and Therapy. Presence 14(2), 119–146 (2005)
47. Rizzolatti, G., Arbib, M.A.: From grasping to speech: imitation might provide a missing link: [Reply]. Trends in Neurosciences 22(4), 52 (1999)
48. Rizzolatti, G., Arbib, M.A.: Language within our grasp. Trends Neurosci. 21, 188–194 (1998)
49. Rogoff, B.: Becoming a Cooperative Parent in a Parent Cooperative. In: Rogoff, B., Goodman Turkanis, C., Bartlett, L. (eds.) Learning Together, Oxford University Press, New York (2001)
50. Rogoff, B.: The cultural nature of human development. Oxford University Press, New York (2003)
51. Rosenbaum, P., King, S., Law, M., King, G., Evans, J.: Family-centered services: A conceptual framework and research review. Physical and Occupational Therapy in Pediatrics 18(1), 1–20 (1998)
52. Schleirmacher, F.: Hermeneutics: The Handwritten Manuscripts. Scholars Press, Missoula, (1977, 1996)
53. Schön, D.: The Reflective Practitioner – How professionals think in action. Basic Books, New York (1983)
54. Schön, D.: Educating the Reflective Practitioner. Josey-Bass, San Francisco (1987)
55. Steels, L.: The Autotelic Principle. In: Iida, F., Pfeifer, R., Steels, L., Kuniyoshi, Y. (eds.) Embodied Artificial Intelligence. LNCS (LNAI), vol. 3139, pp. 231–242. Springer, Heidelberg (2004)
56. Sternberg, R.J.: Handbook of Creativity, 8th edn., Cambridge, New York (2005)
57. Thorpe, W.H.: Learning and Instinct in Animals, 2nd edn. Methuen and Company, London (1963)
58. Varela, F., Thompson, E., Rosch, E.: The embodied mind. MIT, Cambridge (1991)

59. Weiss, P.L., Kedar, R., Shahar, M.: TIES that BIND: An Introduction to Domain Mapping as a Visualization Tool for Virtual Rehabilitation. CyberPsychology and Behavior 9(2), 114–122 (2006)
60. Whiten, A.: Imitation of the Sequential Structure of Actions by Chimpanzees (Pan troglodytes). J. Comp. Psychol. 112, 270–281 (1998)
61. Wood, D.J., Bruner, J.S., Ross, G.: The role of tutoring in problem solving. Journal of Child Psychiatry and Psychology 17(2), 89–100 (1976)
62. Yan, Z., Fischer, K.: Dynamic growth modeling of human cognitive microdevelopment. In: Proc. 2nd International Conference on Development and Learning, pp. 221–227 (2002)

Video examples online at "Sherman56" YouTube

Part III

Technology Acceptance in Medical Decision Support Systems

Chapter 9
Image-Guided Surgery and Its Adoption

Michael Meehan

Knobbe Martens Olson and Bear, 1717 Pennsylvania Ave NW,
Suite 900, Washington, DC
meehan@stanfordalumni.org

Abstract. The past few decades have seen incredible development of technology and systems for image-assisted surgery. Adoption of image-assisted surgical systems by medical practitioners, however, has lagged considerably behind the advances in technology. Whereas this lag in adoption is not an unknown phenomenon when it comes to technological advancement, it is more troubling in the context of patient safety and patient health. With the use of certain image-assisted surgical systems, operative time can be greatly reduced, patients outcomes can be improved, and morbidity and mortality rates can be reduced. The question is then: why aren't the systems being adopted? This chapter discusses a number of issues related to the adoption of surgical trainers and image assisted surgery, including business and reimbursement issues, training issues, and health care liability structures. Examples are taken form the author's own unadopted advances as well as adopted and unadopted systems from other research and business teams.

Keywords: surgical simulation, virtual surgery, image-guided surgery, surgical planning, adoption patterns.

1 A Brief History and Overview of Image Guided Surgery

Technology can be used to improve performance. That is as true in surgery as it is in sports and auto racing. The scalpel and forceps were both invented over 2000 years ago.[1] In 1895, X-ray imaging was invented.[2] In 2004, the FDA approved the first totally-implantable temporary artificial heart, and in 2006 the first totally-implantable permanent artificial heart.[3] With each of these advances, came an improvement in the care of patients and the survivability of illness and injury. For each of these examples, however, there are a numerous medical advances that were not adopted. Although some advances were not adopted because they were not effective, investigation reveals that this is not always the case. Certain advances have not been adopted, even though their efficacy is proved. The question is why some effective advances, some truly improved technologies are adopted by the broad medical community and some are not. This chapter looks at this issue and uses a number of examples, primarily in image-guided surgery, to examine the questions and raise related issues. There are few answers, but perhaps the patterns that are discovered and discussed herein can help elucidate what drives adoption of technology in surgery.

S. Brahnam & L.C. Jain (Eds.): Adv. Comput. Intell. Paradigms in Healthcare 5, SCI 326, pp. 173–188.
springerlink.com

2 A Brief History and Overview of Image Guided Surgery

The field of image guided surgery is considered by some to be just over twenty years old.[4] The advances in image guided surgery are tied in part to technological and scientific improvements in imaging and 3D computer graphics. Looking back into the Technical Report archive at the University of North Carolina, a very well-respected computer graphics and medical imaging program, we see a glimpse of the development of the field of image-guided surgery. The archive has in it, for example, the early work of Mark Levoy, Turner Whitted, Richard Holloway, and Stephen Pizer in the late 1980s.[5] This work looked at new 3D computer graphics rendering techniques, medical imaging, and head-mounted displays.[6], [7], [8] These are some of the building blocks of later image-guided surgery systems built at UNC in the mid 1990s and after.[9]

Image guided surgery may be definable by its use of imaging to aid the surgeon to perform a more effective or more accurate surgery. In some respects, the now-traditional use of ultrasound to guide needles being inserted into the liver for ablation might be considered by some to be image-guided surgery because the images produced by the ultrasound are used by the surgeon to help guide the needle. More likely to be included in any definition of image guided surgery, though, would be the use of pre-operative imaging, such as CT scans, during surgery to help the surgeon plan or execute the surgery. One example of this is Pizer's work at the University of North Carolina in which preoperative CT angiograms are registered with intraoperative fluoroscopy in order to provide the surgeon with a combined image of a region of the body that was not previously possible. This can, for example, enable intraoperative viewing of structures inside the patient that would otherwise be "shaded" by bone during intraoperative fluoroscopy, and therefore not visible intraoperatively to the surgeon. This technology can aid numerous types of surgeries, including percutaneous rhizotomy.[10]

More examples of image-guided surgical systems are discussed in the rest of this chapter. In each case, the advance uses imaging or graphics in a way that was not previously available in order to help the doctor perform more effective surgeries.

3 Unadopted Advances

The advances in image guided surgery that have not been adopted are far too numerous to count and probably outnumber the adopted advances. Researchers and companies are constantly creating new image-guidance technology to improve the medical practice and reduce costs. Some advances even make possible that which was previously impossible. Consider, for example, the work on 3D telepresence for use in remote medical consultation under Dr. Henry Fuchs, of the University of North Carolina.[11] This group has built a system that allows a medical professional that is physically collocated with the patient consult with a medical professional that is remote from the patient. This would be useful on battlefields or geographically isolated medical centers, and would provide patients at remote sites access to medical professionals from all over the world. As of yet, however, this technology has not been adopted.

3.1 Improving Mandibular Distraction

Among the unadopted advances have been some of the author's own research projects. Consider, for example, the author's work at Stanford University in mandibular distraction.[12] Mandibular distraction is a procedure in which bones can be severed or broken and then slowly pulled apart, or distracted, in order to promote growth in the bone. Of course, distracting bone is not as simple as cutting it in two or more pieces, separating those pieces into the desired locations, and merely waiting for the bone in the sutures to grow into place. Bone in a typical adult can grown at a rate of 1mm per day. Therefore, in order to grow the bone, it must be distracted slowly and carefully.

Typically, the mandibular distraction procedure involves attaching the bone to external fixators. These fixators are normally attached to a screw or similar device in order to both secure the bone and control its distraction. After attaching the fixators, the doctor will, on a daily basis, advance the screw in order to lengthen the mandible. Once the mandible has been distracted to its desired length, the fixators will remain in place until the bone is properly formed, after which time they will be removed. This procedure allows restoration of aesthetics and function that were not available previously. Further, similar procedures are performed on many other bones in the human body.

In order to how to distract the mandible, the doctor will normally look to the CT scans and the patient's anatomy in order to determine a desired goal length for the mandible. This is particularly the case when the mandibular deformity is unilateral. When the deformity is unilateral, the doctor can look at the non-deformed side in order to determine a desired length for the deformed side on attempt to mirror the non-deformed side.

The image-guidance system that we built augmented this procedure and allowed it to be planned in ways that were not previously possible. Our system provided improvements in a number of ways. In typical procedures, the there is little more than the surgeon's expertise and reading CT scans, and possibly attempting to mirror the deformed mandible to the non-deformed side, if the deformity is uniform. Further, the doctor can only guess at how the skin and soft tissue will appear after the mandible has been distracted. Our system provides a number of advancements over the traditional, non-image-guided procedure. First, of all, it allows the surgeons to construct the distraction, using a virtual model of the patient. The surgeon can view how the bone would grow and view the outcome of the distraction. This also allows the surgeon to try out and refine more than one distraction path. This is important because distractors distract in a single direction. The location and orientation of the osteotomy and the alignment of the distractor will define the growth path, and thereby, the result of the distraction. Our system allows surgeons to "practice" by performing multiple virtual osteotomies and distractions, and thereby settle on one that results in the desired distraction.[13]

The system takes as input the volumetric CT data and from there performs a marching-cubes analysis in order to determine a 3D model of the bone in the CT data.[14] Once the 3D model is in place, the model is displayed to the surgeon using a 3D rendering on a 2D computer screen. We considered rendering stereoscopically in order to present the data in 3D to the doctor, but this would require specialized hardware, such as a head-mounted display, an alternating-row or alternating-column display or LCD shutter system, etc. If our system required such specialized hardware, we believed, then it would be very unlikely to make it into a doctor's office or workroom. Therefore, in order to increase the likelihood of adoption, we chose a more common configuration: the standard PC. Further, we did not want to require a dedicated PC. Therefore, we developed the system to run on PCs with certain graphics card and memory requirements. Although this may require that a surgeon purchase a new PC in order to use the software, the PC can still be used for the myriad tasks for which PCs are normally employed.

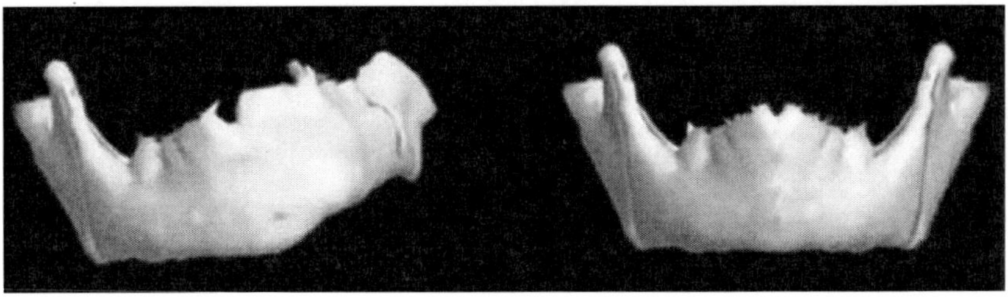

Fig. 1. Deformed mandible (Left) and a mirrored, healthy mandible (Right)

Another manner in which the system improves the traditional procedure is to provide virtual mirroring for the case where the deformity is unilateral. This is depicted in Figure 1. The surgeon provides a mirror line (depicted in Figure 2) and, from there, a mirror of the CT scan is calculated. The algorithm used is a simple axial alignment along the mirror plane and inversion of the coordinates along the axis normal to the mirror plane. The mirrored CT scan is then displayed in ghost, or wireframe in order that the surgeon can see the mirrored CT scan. This provides a great advantage over the non-image-guidance procedure because it provides a "virtual template" or goal for the distraction procedure. With this, the surgeon can perform virtual osteotomies and distractions and see how those distractions will approximate the mirrored, non-deformed jaw.

Our system goes beyond allowing the surgeon to perform multiple, virtual distractions before ever bringing the patient into the operating room. Beyond providing a mirrored CT image of the non-deformed mandible. The system also estimates how the patient will look after the distraction. When the mandible is distracted, the soft tissue, such as muscle, fat, and skin, will compress, stretch, and otherwise react to the changes in the underlying bone. These changes help define the appearance of the patient post-distraction. Our system looks at the structural properties of the soft tissue in order to estimate the appearance of the patient. The soft tissue is estimated using 3D surface scans of the patient and based on the underlying bone from the CT scan. From there, the soft tissue is approximated as a mass and spring model, which is stretched and deformed as the mandible is distracted.[15]

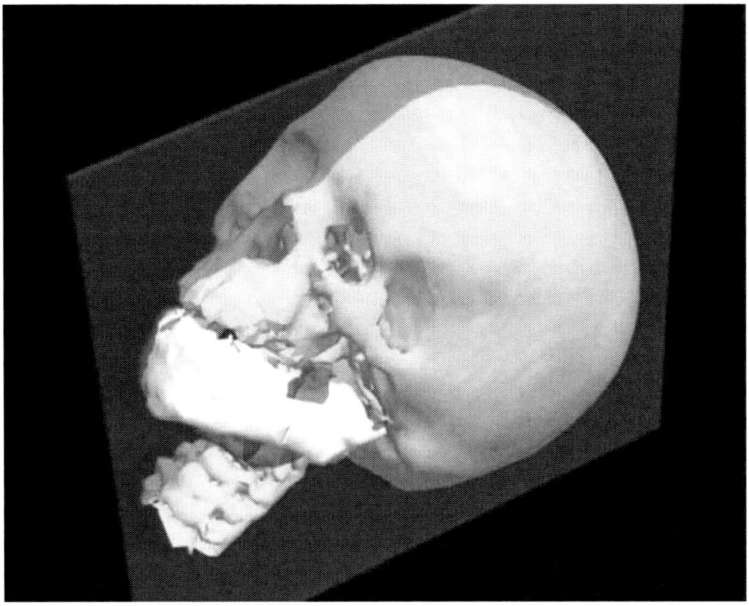

Fig. 2. The surgeon can define a mirror plane (shown in red). The mirror image of the mandible is shown in translucent blue. The existing, deformed mandible is shown in white.

This system was further refined to go beyond merely improving planning of the traditional procedure. Mandibular and other types of distraction rely on linear distractors. Mandibular deformities are not, however, always correctable with linear distraction. Further, it is also possible that a non-linear distraction might produce a better result, even in cases where linear distraction would provide a workable result. As noted above, the furthest a physician will typically distract a bone is 1mm per day. There is another issue with rate of distraction as well. Bone cannot be distracted at too slow a rate. Otherwise, the bone may fuse prematurely. That is, if the bone is distracted too little on a particular day, the fracture may ossify and distraction will cease unless the bone is refractured. Premature fusing is less of an issue in linear distraction because the bone is typically advanced uniformly along the osteotomy. If one were to non-linearly distract a bone, however, then, by definition, different portions of the bone will advance at different rates. Consider the non-linear mandibular distraction pictured in Figure 3. As the mandible is being distracted from P_1 to P_2 along the non-linear path, various portions of the surface of the osteotomy (defined by the normal to the surface of R_1 at P_1 and R_2 at P_2) will travel at different rates. Most intuitively, as the osteotomy placement rounds a curve, the points on the osteotomy on the inside of a curve will cover less distance on a given day and those on the outside of the curve will cover more distance. Therefore, a physician would have to be very careful to avoid both premature ossification and failures due to over-distraction. Figure 4 illustrates this and shows an example of "backtracking," where a portions of the osteotomy would actually have to travel backwards in order to continue on the non-linear osteotomy.

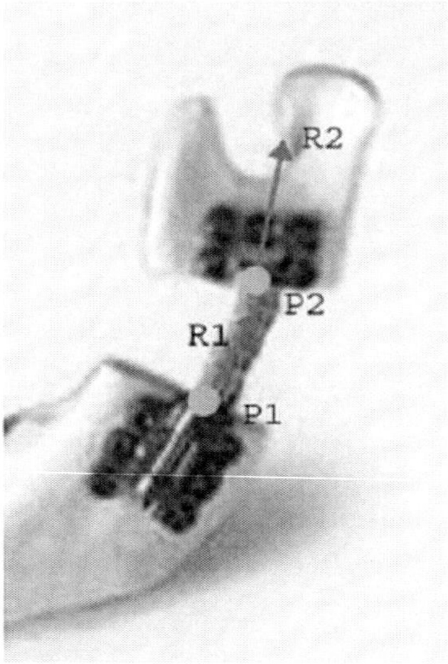

Fig. 3. Non-linear osteotomy

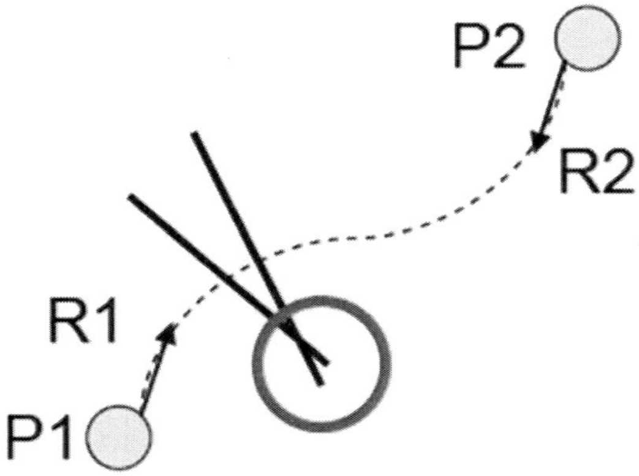

Fig. 4. An example of a collision due to "backtracking." One of multiple issues of concern when performing a non-linear osteotomy.

Our system handles these issues by using an iteratively-defined Hermite curve and performing a step-by-step analysis and analyzing the points on the osteotomy at each time step and flagging or otherwise prohibiting over-advancement, under-advancement, and backtracking.[16] The Hermite curve is parametrically defined as

$$p(t)=(2t^3-3t^2+1)P_1 +(-2t^3+3t^2)P_2 + (t^3-2t^2+t)R_1+(t^3-t^2)R_2$$

If there is a violation of the distraction constraints, then the normals used to define the Hermite curve are adjusted, with the normal closer to the constraint violation being distracted. This flattens the curve in the region of the constraint violation, while still maintaining a smooth curve. The system can output the non-linear distraction in a manner that would allow a physical non-linear distractor to be machined.

Notwithstanding the significant advances that this system represents, it allows for better guidance and prediction of results as well as allowing the creation of non-linear distraction plans that might not otherwise be possible, this technology still has not been adopted. Another example of a non-adopted system is given below. Later I discuss possible reasons for the non-adoption of these advancements.

3.2 Preoperative Craniosynostosis Planning

Another example of an unadopted medical imaging advance that could drastically improve surgical care and save money is the work of my research group, under the direction of Dr. Sabine Girod, at Stanford University, which is related to the work of Clijmans et al., in which a preoperative surgical plan for craniosynostosis is developed using 3D imaging.[17], [18] Craniosynostosis is a condition in which in which a baby's skull forms improperly. At birth, the human skull is normally made up of 45 separate bones attached by fibrous membranes called "sutures." As a baby grows, the sutures between bones close, resulting in larger pieces of bone. This suture closure will typically result in the formation of approximately 28 bones by early adulthood. If some of these sutures close prematurely, then, as the child's brain grows, it may not have enough room to expand. This may lead to increased intracranial pressure, asymmetry of the face, malocclusion, and, in some cases, strabismus.[19]

Surgery is used to correct the prematurely-formed sutures. The surgery is not as simple as merely performing osteotomies at the sites of the prematurely fused sutures. In order to properly correct a child's skull, the surgeon separates pieces of the skull and relocates those pieces. The separated pieces of bone are reshaped on the child's head, often in a significantly altered configuration. The surgeon may use plates, screws, and surgical sutures to hold the pieces in place. The scalp is then replaced over the reshaped skull. The various varieties of these operations can take 3-7 hours depending on complexity. As is easy to imagine, the operations takes such a long time not only because of the actual process of cutting and replacing the skull bones, but also because of the complex 3D nature of the problem.

In both the "Clijmans" and our group's systems ("the Girod system"), much of the operative planning can happen before the operation and that operative plan can be taken into the operating room. In both systems, the surgeon can import CT scans of the patient's skull, and the system will allow the surgeon to manipulate the virtual skull, performing osteotomies and reconfiguring the pieces of bone. The surgeon can then view the reassembled skull in the 3D imaging system. Unlike in conventional craniosynostosis surgeries, surgeons can try multiple operative plans using the preoperative planning systems of Girod and Clijmans. That is, the surgeon can make a plan for the osteotomies of the child's skull bones and for placement of the separated bones to reform the shape of a child's skull. The surgeon can view a realistic estimate of the appearance of the planned placement using 3D visualization to view the bones themselves. The surgeon may also be able to view an estimate of how the child will look by looking at a soft tissue simulation of the face and skull on top of the replaced bones. If the doctor does not like this placement of the bones, then she can hit the reset button and work on a new plan for the placement of the bones. This type of "second try" is not available in traditional surgery. A surgeon cannot simply hit a reset button and undue osteotomies actually performed on a living patient in order to obtain a better placement or better end result.

The operative plans developed by the surgeons using either of these systems can be taken into the operating room. In Girod's system, graphical visualization is used to bring the system into the operating room. The real surgical instruments are tracked during the operation, as is the child's head (and thereby his skull). The planned osteotomies are seen on a monitor and a surgeon can guide the surgical instruments into the correct place in order to follow the plan. Clijmans' system, on the other hand, allows the surgeon to make surgical guides or templates out of aluminum or plastic foil. The surgeon can bring these guides or templates into the operating room in order to execute the planned osteotomies.

For both systems, the surgical times for various craniosynostosis surgeries can be reduced drastically when compared to similar surgeries performed without preoperative planning. The surgeon will have to spend time developing the plan ahead of time, but the time in the operating room can be reduced by 40%-50%.[20] In the surgeries reported in Clijmans' work, the planning phase of the operation is likely to take at least as much time as the time saved in the operating room. Further the panning stage can take much longer if multiple plans are investigated. This may mean that the doctor may end up spending as much or more time that she otherwise would have in traditional surgery. It is important to note, however, that operative time and surgeon time are not equivalent. Top surgeons may get paid an annual rate that works out to a few hundred dollars per hour (including operating and non-operating hours). Operating rooms, however, may cost as much as a hundred dollars per *minute*. A surgeon's time is not an infinitely-available commodity, but in terms of raw cost, it is far cheaper to have a surgeon spend a few hours in preparation in order to reduce a craniofacial surgery from four hours down to two hours. The net fiscal savings is likely to be a net savings of around $10k for the hospital for a single surgery.

Money is not the only savings, though, and perhaps is not the most important. It is generally accepted that, other things being equal, operative time is proportional to both morbidity rate, the rate of infection or other side effects caused by surgery, and mortality rate, the rate of death due to operations.[21] The reduced morbidity and mortality are certainly appealing aspects to the patients, their families, the hospitals, and the doctors, but they also help society at large. Although clearly very valuable, it is hard to quantify the benefit to a patient or their family due to the reduced chance of morbidity and mortality. It might be possible, however, to quantify the saving to society the reduction of morbidity and mortality. In a purely economic sense, a reduced mortality rate would increase the expected value of the amount of money a person would make during their lifetime. A person can expect to make $1 million to $2 million in their lifetime, depending on education level.[22] All other benefits aside, reducing mortality rate of craniosynostosis surgery by a mere 1% would increase the nation's cumulative GDP over that person's lifetime by $10k - $20k. Although much harder to predict, reduced morbidity rates would also produce some savings in terms of reduced health care rates.

3.3 Issues in the Non-adoption

Given the clear savings and benefits that these preoperative planning systems provide, it is a wonder why they are not used in standard practice. It is true that some of the savings are hard to quantify. From the above discussion, it is clear that is would be difficult to estimate or quantify the savings to society of the reduced operative times provided by the image-guided craniosynostosis surgery planning systems or the improved functionality provided by the mandibular planning system. The increase in quality of life of the patients and their families due to reduced morbidity and mortality are of high value, certainly, but are also fairly unquantifiable. The reduction of mortality and morbidity rate would be of great economic value to society, but there is no data on what percentage reduction in to quantify how much the reduced operative increases productivity as measured by lifetime salary.

Some cost savings associated with using the pre-operative planning systems are more certain. There are the monetary savings discussed above due to the reduced operative times, saving $10k by reducing a four hour operation by 40%-50%. If the planning system costs $100k, for example, then it would pay for itself in ten operations. And since these systems may be useful for multiple types of operations, it is easy to imagine that they would pay for themselves within a few months, if not a few weeks.

What, then, has caused the systems to not be used in operating rooms? In the final section of this chapter is a discussion of the effect that introducing a new operative process can have on adoption of a new surgical system. This is most clearly illustrated by contrasting adopted and unadopted advances, and is therefore left for later discussion. But what else might be causing the non-adoption of these systems?

Medical devices must be approved by the FDA in order to be marketed and sold. Typically, doctors can get institution-internal approval to test equipments in the operating room. In order to sell the equipment, however, the selling company must have FDA approval for any device sold. If there has been a similar device approved by the FDA previously, then the company can apply for an equivalence application for the device, called a 501(k) application. If the device is not equivalent to anything that has come before, then a new Premarket Approval (PMA) application must be submitted. The requirements for either of these applications are stringent and complex, but for the purposes of this chapter, it is important to note the cost. The cost to simply file a 510(k) is $2k -$4k, depending on the size of your company. The fees for filing a PMA application start at $54k for small companies and climb to over $200k for large companies.[23] There are additionally direct and lost costs of the FDA application process. Electronic medical devices must pass, for example, UL testing, and the medical device companies often need to hire lawyers or other consultants in order to get the device through the FDA. It is difficult to estimate the cost for FDA approval, but it is certain to be tens or hundreds of thousands of dollars at a minimum, even for device-equivalence 510(k) applications.

In addition, the economics of hospitals is such that mere FDA approval and usefulness is not enough to get a device into a hospital and in general use. Without insurance company reimbursement, doctors are unlikely to use a new technology and patients are unlikely to demand it (and pay for it). Insurance companies make their own decisions as to the use of which medical devices are approved for reimbursement, and this decision will usually come after the device has been approved by the FDA. For example, the FDA approved the now-ubiquitous magnetic resonance imaging (MRI) machine in March 1984. Ten months later, the Blue Cross Blue Shield still considered it "premature to accept MRI as a standard, clinically effective, diagnostic technique even for general applications to the central nervous system." In June 1985, Blue Cross Blue Shield approved reimbursement for certain uses of MRI. Further, it was not until November 1995 that the Health Care Financing Administration, which oversees Medicare, approved the MRI for coverage reimbursement.[24]

The monetary road for a medical device company is a difficult one. In a good case, the medical device company may have developed a useful equivalent of an existing device, and, even after spending hundreds of thousands of dollars developing the device, spend another fifty to one hundred thousand dollars getting the device approved by the FDA. Thereafter, they must convince the hospitals to buy the device. The company must do so in the face of the hospitals taking on the legal liability responsibility for the standard of care being administered. Once the device is successfully sold to hospitals, then insurance companies must be convinced that the device should be reimbursed as a generally accepted standard of care – as it is very unlikely that the insurance companies will approve something for use before it is in regular use in hospitals.

With all of these monetary difficulties facing companies that make medical devices, it is clear that the medical device companies will need considerable wherewithal, in terms of time, resources, and money, to go through the long process of getting the device approved by the FDA, into hospitals, getting doctors trained, and getting health care reimbursement. Having enough reserves and enough time may be less of an issue for large companies such as Johnson and Johnson, Stryker, and General Electric, but it is often be beyond the meager budgets of start-ups and research labs.

4 Adopted Advances

There are a number of technological advancements that have made their way into operating rooms. As noted above, MRIs were not approved for insurance reimbursement for over a year after FDA approval, and then only for certain medical indications.[25] Many technologies are not adopted that quickly. Laparoscopy, which is now widely used in many forms, was under various stages of development for hundreds of years before it was used in operating rooms. Nezhat notes that "almost all elements necessary to make the endoscope viable existed [in the year 1710]."[26] From there, it took over 200 years, until the 1980s until any of the forms of laparoscopy were incorporated into training for residents.[27] It was only in the 1990s that the Society of Laparoscopic Surgeons was formed.[28] After the lengthy courtship with the medical profession, laparoscopic procedures are now generally considered to be the preferred method of treatment among alternative surgical procedures.

Another more recent advance in image-guided surgery is the work of a small North Carolina start-up, InnerOptic Technology, Inc. InnerOptic has built a system that allows surgeons to view, in 3D on an auto-stereoscopic screen, ultrasound, ablation, and guidance data. In traditional surgery, when a surgeon attempts to ablate, or burn, a tumor in a liver, the surgeon opens up the patient and locates the tumor using ultrasound visualization. Once the tumor is located, the surgeon attempts to drive an ablation needle into the tumor. The surgeon can check to see if the needle is correctly located by moving the ultrasound wand and looking at the ultrasound image and attempting to determine from the image whether the needle is correctly placed with respect to the tumor. The task takes a great deal of skill and surgeons will often have to drive the ablation needle into the tumor multiple times before the needle is properly located within the tumor. These multiple needle drives do additional damage to the liver and take additional operative time.

InnerOptic's InVision system is used in the operating room and tracks the positions and orientations of the ablation needle and the ultrasound wand during the ablation procedure. The system takes in the position data and provides an image of the ablation needle relative to the ultrasound image. The system also provides guidance data for the needle with respect to the ultrasound image. The result is that the doctor can see how the needle is being driven with respect to the ultrasound image, and thereby the tumor. The system will even display a projection line that will show where the needle will enter the ultrasound image if the surgeon drives the needle in a straight line. The surgeon can line up the graphically-projected driving line of the ablation needle and drive the needle to the tumor that the surgeon spotted in the ultrasound image. InnerOptic has had great interest from surgeons. Further, they have performed tests and report a drastic increase in accuracy of striking the tumor with the needle, from 66% accuracy rate with the traditional ultrasound-only method, to 92% with their InVision System. The study also showed that surgeon were able to successfully drive the needle to the tumor in 70% less time. They have recently received FDA approval, and hope to soon have their system adopted by surgeons in operating rooms.[29]

These examples are all clearly important technological advances that have already been adopted, or in the case of the InnerOptic InVision system, appear to be well into the process of being adopted. The question is, then, why are some of the technological advances adopted and others are not? The next section discusses these issues and discusses

5 Contrasting Adoption and Non-adoption

What drives the adoption of one technology and opposes the adoption of another? The answer to this question cannot be simply profit. It is true that a company that gets its technologies adopted is going to be more profitable, and academics that get their technologies adopted are going to gain fame, and possibly money. But profit is not the only thing. Society, generally speaking, gives money for things that it values. And the same is the case here. If a technology is adopted in the operating room, regardless of the profit granted the technology's creator, it is because it improves the operation in some way. That improvement can be through temporal efficiency, which, all other things being equal, usually has coupled with it monetary savings, reduced chance of infection, and freeing of resources. Additionally, in some cases, as noted above, the technology makes possible operations that were not previously.

The economics of the adoption of new technologies makes taking an idea to a developed and accepted product difficult, as discusses above. The costs and time involved may be more than many research institution and small companies can afford. The economics is clearly an important factor to non-adoption, but it may not be the only one. There may also be a pattern emerging from a few of the examples herein that relates to the type of change in process or surgical procedure that is needed in order to adopt the new technology.

Comparing the changes in surgical procedure and process necessitated by the image-guidance systems developed by our and Clijmans' teams with that necessitated by the InVision system developed by InnerOptic, we see a stark contrast in what the surgeon will need to learn in order to use the system. To simplify the discussion of craniosynostosis above, in traditional craniosynostosis surgery, the surgeon enters the operating room, cuts back the scalp, dissects the skull, removes the bones, and replaces the skull bones in a different configuration to improve symmetry and spacing. Using, for example, the system built by Girod et al., the surgeon will first spend time in front of a computer system, develop a plan for the dissection and reconfiguration of the skull bones, that system will be imported into a imaging system in the operation room, the surgeon then views the output of the operating room system in order to find and dissect the bones based on the plan, and similarly interacts with the image-guidance system in order to place the dissected bones based on the original plan. The general sequence of steps needed for our mandibular distraction system are parallel, requiring preoperative planning and intraoperative guidance to enact the preoperative mandibular plan.

To simplify the traditional ablation procedure, the surgeon finds a tumor using ultrasound imaging, drives the ablation needle into a tumor based primarily on hand-eye coordination and experience, she can check to see whether the needle is correctly driven by looking for the needle in the ultrasound image, and then she ablates the tumor using microwave radiation emitted by the needle. Using InnerOptic's InVision system, the surgeon still determines the location of tumors based on the ultrasound image, she still drives the ablation needle to the tumor, but instead guides the needle using the imaging of the projected needle in addition to her hand-eye coordination, and once she checks with the ultrasound wand that the needle has been correctly driven, she ablates the tumor.

Both of these technologies, pre-operative planning for craniosynostosis and image-guidance for ablation procedures, represent great advances in treatment. The craniosynostosis systems allow for preoperative planning and re-planning that is simply not possible in the traditional surgery. They also greatly reduce operative time, which has commensurate reductions in cost and morbidity and mortality. InnerOptic's needle ablation system allows for greatly increased accuracy in driving ablation needle, thereby reducing damage to healthy portions of the liver and reducing operative time.

In contrasting the discussed technological advances, however, one sees an important distinction. The craniosynostosis systems require new stages in the procedure, namely the preoperative planning at a computer workstation and intraoperative guidance based on that plan. The mandibular distraction planning system also requires new, preoperative planning steps and intraoperative guidance. In contrast, the InVision system at least from the perspective of the surgeon, simply provides new information to the surgeon – it does not replace of any part of the traditional procedure. A surgeon could use the ultrasound wand and the ablation needle provided with the InVision system without necessarily having to even consider the additional information presented on the screen by the InVision system, such as the drive projection of the ablation needle. The surgeon could simply look at the output of the ultrasound and rely on her hand-eye coordination in order to drive the needle to the tumor. In fact, in all likelihood a surgeon who was learning to use the InVision system could both rely on her hand-eye coordination and look at the new information on the drive projection of the needle.

The approach of the InVision system is to take a small step forward in information and procedure and allow the surgeon to rely on her previous skill and knowledge in order to perform the procedure. Our systems, on the other hand, require new skills and new types of interaction with new types of equipment. Certainly any surgeon can learn the skills necessary for adopting a new procedure. But when can they learn to use the new systems? In the abstract, before the surgeon is trained on the new equipment, the surgeon may forego the use of the new equipment during any given operation in order to not jeopardize the quality of care. When, then, will the surgeon get real-world experience using the new system? If the surgeon is not trained on the system, then it seems unlikely that her hospital would ever adopt the new technique as a standard procedure. Further, if surgeons and hospitals are not performing surgeries using the systems, then it is also unlikely that insurance companies will adopt the new procedure as a reimbursable standard of care. Until something is a reimbursable standard of care, it will be difficult to get broad adoption of the procedure or the equipment.

Applying this proposition to the InVision system, we see that it fares better. Since the system can be used by a surgeon for additional information during an existing operation, should be much easier to integrate into the medical establishment. Surgeons will be able to use it without affecting the standard of care because they will continue to have all of the previously-available information and can seamlessly switch between the traditional method and viewing the new information. Therefore, the surgeon will be able to progress with current standard of care and incorporate new information at whatever pace is comfortable. Eventually, the new information, the new procedure, if it is better for the surgeon, will be adopted by the hospitals and insurance companies as the new standard of care.

Returning to our and Clijmans' image-guidance systems, new information is available – the preoperative plans for dissection and replacement of the skull bones. If the surgeon does not feel comfortable guiding the scalpel based on the preoperative plan, however, then she is, essentially, reverting back to the traditional surgical technique. The same is true if she is not comfortable reconfiguring the dissected skull based on the preoperative plan. If the doctor reverts to the traditional system and does not use the preoperative plan for either dissection or reconfiguration of the dissected skull bones, then she is likely to feel that she wasted her time in creating the preoperative plan, and this can be hours in an already busy surgical week. If the preoperative plan reduces hours in the operating room, then the hours making the preoperative plan may well be worthwhile. If the plan is not used, however, then the time planning is essentially lost.

That is not to say that there is never room for a drastically new procedure or technology. As noted above, the MRI was adopted by insurance companies for some indications within two years of its FDA approval. This was a new machine, parallel to and separate from X-ray and other imaging technologies that already existed at the time. Further, and perhaps a closer parallel to the tumor ablation, mandibular distraction, and craniosynostosis systems, laparoscopic surgery was eventually adopted, even though it took hundreds of years since its first consideration and decades after it was commercially available for it to become the standard of care. The laparoscopic procedures required the surgeons to learn and adopt drastically-different procedures for numerous surgical procedures. Even though the laparoscopic versions of the procedures reduced trauma and, in some cases, operative time, the medical community did not adopt the procedures with open arms and hearts. In fact, as recently as the 1990s, many surgeons still criticized laparoscopic surgery as overused and laparoscopic surgeons as opportunistic.[30]

Of course, one can never make sweeping generalizations that hold true in every case. Perhaps, however, these examples of adopted and unadopted image-guidance technologies teach us something both as technologist wishing to help another field and businesspeople wishing to choose a good product to pursue for our business. It seems that in addition to needing the economic and temporal wherewithal to develop a medical device, one path to improved adoptability is to make a product that provides the doctor an opportunity to maintain the existing standard of care while getting more information from the new system. This would allow the doctor can easily maintain the current standard of care while learning to use the new information presented by the image-guidance system and thereby improving the standard of care.

References

1. Willey, D.: Roman period surgery set on show, BBC News (December 10, 2007), `http://news.bbc.co.uk/2/hi/europe/7137224.stm`
2. Peters, P., Roentgen, W.C., the Discovery of X-rays: Textbook of Radiology, `http://www.medcyclopaedia.com/library/radiology`
3. American Heart Association, Artificial Heart, `http://www.americanheart.org/presenter.jhtml?identifier=4444`
4. Galloway, R., Peters, T.: Image-Guided Interventions, p. 1. Springer, Heidelberg (2007)
5. University of North Carolina Computer Science, Technical Report Archive, `http://cs.unc.edu/Research/tech-report.html`
6. Levoy, M., Whitted, T.: The Use of Points as a Display Primitive, UNC Technical Report Archive, TR85-022 (1985)
7. Gauch, J.M., Oliver, W.R., Pizer, S.M.: Multiresolution Shape Descriptions and Their Applications in Medical Imaging, UNC Technical Report Archive, TR87-018 (1987)
8. Holloway, R.L.: Head-Mounted Display Technical Report, UNC Tech-nical Report Archive, TR87-015 (1987)
9. Liu, A., Bullitt, E., Pizer, S.M.: Surgical Instrument Guidance Using Synthesized Anatomical Structures, UNC Technical Report Archive, TR96-045 (1996)
10. Percutaneous rhizotomy is a procedure to sever the spinal nerve to relieve pain. Gauch, note 7
11. 3D Telepresence for Medical Consultation, `http://www.cs.unc.edu/Research/nlm`
12. Meehan, M., Morris, D., Maurer, C.R., Antony, A.K., Barbagli, F., Salisbury, K., Girod, S.: Virtual 3D Planning and Guidance of Mandibular Distraction Osteo-genesis, vol. 1256, pp. 382–388 (June 2003)
13. Meehan et al, note 12, p. 382
14. Lorensen, W., Cline, H.: Marching cubes: A high resolution 3d surface construction algorithm. Computer Graphics 21(4), 163–169 (1987)
15. Teschner, M., Girod, S., Girod, B.: Realistic modeling of elasto-mechanical properties of soft tissue and its evaluation. Computer Assisted Radiology and Surgery, vol. 1230, pp. 51–56 (2001)
16. Foley, J.D., van Dam, A., Feiner, S.K., Hughes, J.F.: Computer Graphics: Principles and Practice, 2nd edn. Addison Wesley, Reading (1987)
17. Girod, S., et al.: Computer-aided 3-D simulation and prediction of cra-niofacial surgery: a new approach. Journal of Maxillofacial Surgery 29(3), 156–158 (2001)
18. Clijmans, T., et al.: Computer supported pre-operative planning of craniofa-cial surgery: from patient to template. In: IFMBE proceedings 3rd European medical & biological engineering conference, Prague, Czech Republic, vol. 11 (November 2005)

19. Kabbani, H., Raghuveer, T.S.: Craniosynostosis. American Family Physician 69(12), 2863–2870 (2004-06-15)
20. Clijmans, note 18
21. Scheer, A., et al.: Laparoscopic Colon Surgery: Does Operative Time Matter? Diseases of the Colon & Rectum 52(10), 1746–1752 (2009)
22. Thompson, M.: Earnings of a Lifetime: Comparing Women and Men with College and Graduate Degrees. Context 10, 2 (2009)
23. FDA, Overview of Medical Devices, The FDA estimates that its costs for actually reviewing these applica-tions are $18k for 510(k) applications and $870k for PMA applications. Govern-ment Accountability Office, Report to Congressional Addressees: Medical Devices (January 2009), `http://www.fda.gov/MedicalDevices/DeviceRegulationandGuidance/Overview/default.htm`
24. McGivney, Approval Processes Different for Devices and Drugs, Physician Executive (July 1990)
25. McGivney, note 24
26. Nezhat, Let There Be Light: A Historical Analysis of Endoscopy's Ascen-sion Since Antiquity, ch. 4 (2005)
27. Nezhat, note 26, ch. 23
28. Nezhat, note 26, ch. 24
29. InnerOptic Technology, Inc., `http://www.inneroptic.com`
30. Nezhat, note 26, ch. 24

Chapter 10
The Role of Presence in Healthcare Technology Applications

Paul Skalski

School of Communication, Cleveland State University, 2121 Euclid Ave., Cleveland, OH 44115, USA
p.skalski@csuohio.edu

Abstract. This chapter addresses the role of presence or "the perceptual illusion of nonmediation" [26] in user responses to technologies for healthcare, with particular attention to intelligent decision support systems (IDSS). It begins by defining presence and reviewing relevant research on presence-related responses to agents, virtual reality systems, and other technologies. It then discusses the implications of presence to researchers and health practitioners with an interest in IDSS, including a series of recommendations.

Keywords: Presence, telepresence, virtual reality, agents, new media technologies.

1 Introduction

When people talk about virtual reality (VR), agents, and other new forms of media, they often mention how the technologies give users a sensation of "being there" in a media environment or "being with" mediated others. These types of reactions to media technologies are now being focused on by scholars interested in the concept of *presence* (or *telepresence*), defined as "the perceptual illusion of non-mediation" [26]. Many aspects of technology contribute to presence. VR technology, for example, typically provides users with more sensory information and interface options than other types of media [4]. Through head-mounted displays, data gloves, and other forms of sensorimotor engagement, VR makes users feel "in" virtual environments (i.e, *spatial presence*). As another example, social agents are computer software programs that exhibit intelligence and can interact with people socially [33]. By exhibiting such human behavior, agents can make users feel "with" virtual others (i.e., *social presence*). Understanding the psychological side of VR and agent experiences through presence and related concepts has tremendous value for both researchers and practitioners with an interest in technologies for health.

This chapter discusses the role of presence in responses to healthcare technologies, with special attention to intelligent decision support systems (IDSS). IDSS

S. Brahnam & L.C. Jain (Eds.): Adv. Comput. Intell. Paradigms in Healthcare 5, SCI 326, pp. 189–200.
springerlink.com

are a broad class of technologies (including forms of VR and agents) that use artificial intelligence techniques to support decision making [38]. In the health field, IDSS can help medical professionals and patients in a number of important ways, such as in making diagnoses and deciding between preventive care options. Few (if any) attempts have been made to connect IDSS to presence, however, despite natural overlaps between the two literatures. This chapter defines presence and reviews research on presence-related responses to technologies used in healthcare, chiefly VR and agents. It then discusses implications of the concept of presence to researchers and health practitioners with an interest in IDSS, including a series of recommendations.

2 (Tele)Presence: An Overview

The term *telepresence* comes from Marvin Minsky, who in 1980 used it to refer to the manipulation of remote objects through technology. In the 1990s, a number of scholars picked up on the concept to help describe what was happening to people in response to emerging media technologies such as VR [10]. At this time, Byron Reeves [30] focused attention on the feeling of "being there" that can be created by advanced media technologies. Jonathan Steuer [36] wrote about dimensions of technology (vividness and interactivity) determining telepresence, while Thomas Sheridan [32] shortened the concept to "presence" and used it to refer to feelings people have while immersed in virtual environments. VR was the subject of a book by Frank Biocca and Mark Levy [6] that discussed the potential for "goggles and gloves" technologies to immerse media users. And two years later, perhaps the most seminal work on presence was published, an explication of the concept by Matthew Lombard and Theresa Ditton [26] that inspired Lombard to start an organization devoted to inquiry into the concept.

This organization, known as the International Society for Presence Research (ISPR), endeavored to define presence as a group and settled on it being "a psychological state or subjective perception in which even though part or all of an individual's current experience is generated by and/or filtered through human-made technology, part or all of the individual's perception fails to accurately acknowledge the role of the technology in the experience" [20]. In the first decade of the 21st century, scholars spent considerable time identifying and studying more specific forms of the concept, including involvement, immersion, social richness, and co-presence [10]. However, the two most commonly researched types have been *spatial presence* or feeling "in" a media environment [41], and *social presence* or feeling "with" mediated others [5]. A third type of presence gaining traction is *self presence*, or experiencing a representation of oneself (such as an avatar) as part of oneself inside a virtual environment [23]. In conjunction with working on conceptualizations of presence, researchers have also worked to identify causes and effects of the perception of non-mediation.

3 Determinants of Presence in Mediated Environments

When considering perception in natural environments with no mediated component, the concept of presence and what creates the feeling of "being there" is generally taken for granted: "I am here, in my environment, so I naturally feel present in this environment." The possibilities are limited to the experience of physical surroundings [36]. However, when ones tries to distinguish the experiences of individuals in natural environments from those in mediated environments, understanding what it means to feel present and what creates that feeling of presence becomes a more important issue. Characteristics of the individual as well as those of different media technologies and content interact to determine the manner in which presence is experienced in different environments.

3.1 Technological Characteristics and Presence

As mentioned, Steuer [36] claims that the vividness and interactivity found in a medium help to evoke telepresence. *Vividness* refers to the technology's ability to produce a rich sensory environment, while *interactivity* refers to the technology's capacity to enable the user to influence the form and content of an environment. The vividness of an environment is defined by the manner in which information is presented to the senses. A vivid medium is one that is high in breadth (the number of sensory channels simultaneously activated) and depth (the degree of resolution within each sensory channel). Conventional media like print, radio and television send signals to only the auditory and/or visual channels and therefore have limited breadth. Newer media such as video games try to supplement this by activating the haptic system and basic orienting systems (those controlling body equilibrium). Some have gone so far as to engage taste and smell systems [28], though this is generally rare.

A medium with great depth delivers more information or data through each sensory channel. For example, the bandwidth and transmission capabilities of a computer showing a YouTube video provide considerably less information to the senses of sight and hearing than a large screen TV showing a high definition Blu-Ray video. A number of studies support the notion that media formal features such as screen size and screen resolution increase presence [25, 8]. Steuer [36] suggests that breadth and depth interact to create the sense of telepresence, and that simultaneous activation of multiple sensory systems can produce a strong feeling of telepresence even when signal depth is low.

An interactive medium is one that provides the user with the ability to alter the form and content of the mediated environment. According to Steuer [36], interactivity is greatly influenced by three factors: *speed* (the time required for the environment to respond to input), *range* (the number of environmental attributes that can be manipulated and the amount of alternatives available for each attribute changed), and *mapping* (how closely actions represented in the virtual environment match the natural actions used to change a real environment). Recent research has shown that mapping in particular positively affects presence, with more mapped interfaces leading to greater presence [34]. In general, real-time interaction where the user performs natural actions that instantaneously alter a wide variety of characteristics in the mediated environment should create a high sense of presence. However, since presence is a psychological state, some users may be more affected than others. In other words, characteristics of a media user also impact presence.

3.2 Individual Differences in Experiencing Presence

Although most attempts to identify determinants of telepresence deal with characteristics of media, attempts have been made to determine characteristics of *individuals* that affect this experience. Along with fitness, alertness, and ability to focus attention, Witmer and Singer [40] consider a person's tendency to identify with characters in stories, sports or video games as a predictor of experienced telepresence. Lombard and Ditton [26] cite willingness to suspend disbelief and knowledge of and prior experience with a medium as important predictors of susceptibility. As part of their MEC model of spatial presence, Wirth et al. [41] include a number of user characteristics potentially impacting presence, including domain specific interest, or how much a person cares about a type of content (such as a film genre). Whitbred, Skalski, Bracken, and Lieberman [39] recently found that receiver apprehension or general unwillingness to attend to communication had a negative impact on presence. Clearly, there are many individual difference variables that may impact the extent to which a person experiences presence, and these should be taken into account in designing and implementing presence-inducing technologies for different populations.

3.3 Content Determinants of Telepresence

A final, understudied cause of presence is *media content*. Whereas research on technology addresses how media form or the manner in which information is delivered makes a person present, the message itself is also important. Lombard and Ditton [26] suggest that social realism (or how realistic a presentation seems in terms of characters, storyline, etc.), use of media conventions (such as on-screen graphics), and the nature of a task presented can all affect the extent to which a person feels presence. Recent research supports the idea that content matters to presence [e.g., 9].

One content feature that has received scant attention from presence researchers is artificial intelligence, which has obvious implications for the design of IDSS for healthcare. Artificial intelligence has been the basis for many medical diagnosis systems [29]. The more artificial intelligence an IDSS exhibits, the greater the social presence a user should feel, since intelligent interactions are a norm of daily life. The Computers As Social Actors (CASA) studies of Reeves and Nass [31] reveal how human beings, as a function of evolution, are hard-wired to treat machines as people, especially when they exhibit human-like characteristics such as intellect. Biocca, Harms and Burgoon [5] furthermore suggest that one of the keys to fully experiencing social presence is a sense of access to another intelligence. It may be, however, that too much intelligence detracts from social presence, if it goes far beyond what would be expected from a human. If so, then artificial intelligence may have a curvilinear effect on presence. Future work on IDSS for healthcare should explore this linkage.

4 Presence and Mediated Healthcare

Most presence scholars in communication, psychology, and related fields are not just interested in presence as an outcome of media exposure, but also in how presence may impact further outcomes of interest in particular domains of study, including entertainment, persuasion, and health, the focus of this chapter. Advanced, presence-inducing technologies have been used for healthcare in a number of ways. As Lombard [24] notes, presence principles are currently being used for e-health purposes such as distance surgery, remote medical care, rehabilitation, and phobia treatment, to name a few. A handful of studies to date have explored the relationship between presence and health technology use outcomes. These may be divided into health studies using (1) VR and (2) agents and other technologies.

4.1 Health Research on VR Technology and Presence

One of the first research initiatives to address the relationship between presence and health outcomes is the EMMA (Engaging Media for Mental Health Applications) project [1]. The goal of the EMMA project has been to investigate how presence-inducing VR technologies may be used for non-addictive, mood stabilizing experiences. Through understanding the relationship between presence and emotions, the researchers hope to develop "mood devices" providing innovative ways of coping with distressing emotions, such as affective, anxiety, and adjustment disorders, and restricted mobility.

Cognitive rehabilitation has also been examined. Castelnuovo et al. [12] have looked into the potential for VR technology to help individuals with traumatic brain injuries. This research has been concerned with testing the added value of VR over traditional approaches to assessment and rehabilitation of cognitive functions. In this research, the core characteristics of a virtual environment that make it useful for mental health applications have been assessed by measuring presence.

In a more targeted, applied study, Brown, Nunez, and Blake [11] created a VR environment to provide nutritional information to HIV positive women in South Africa. Specifically, the environment was a house in which users interacted with others for social support, while also learning about food groups and cleanliness/hygiene issues. Participants in the study who navigated through this high presence-inducing VR system found it usable and enjoyable. Despite finding the amount of information lacking, they thought the information was of high quality, leading the authors to ultimately conclude that this type of system is a useful way to disseminate medical knowledge.

Finally, a number of clever, innovative VR and health studies have been conducted by Jeremy Bailenson and colleagues. This research calls attention to the potential for VR technology to not only replicate real-world experiences but also to surpass them. Bailenson et al. [3], for example, investigated aspects of presence-inducing VR technology that are unique from a media interactivity standpoint, including the ability to capture and review physical behavior and the ability to see an avatar rendered in real time from third-person point of view. Two studies were conducted that allowed users to either learn Tai Chi through viewing a video of an instructor (traditional method) or through seeing a captured image (avatar) of themselves doing moves next to the instructor doing moves, as if they were performing the actions together (VR method). Learning was better in the VR conditions, showing the potential for self-presence inducing VR to serve as a tool for such health applications as physical therapy and exercise.

In related follow-up research, Fox and Bailenson [14] further examined health applications of self presence-inducing VR technology. They conducted three studies testing how virtual representations of the physical self affected exercise behaviors. Specifically, they made realistic avatars of study participants do things like gain weight and perform exercise and found that participants exposed to such avatars (versus control conditions) were significantly more likely to exercise themselves. In another study, Fox and Bailenson [15] focused specifically on presence (an untested assumption in some of this research) and avatar eating. Participants were shown photorealistic avatars of themselves eating healthy and unhealthy foods in a virtual world, to see how it would affect their real-life eating. Results were moderated by sex, with men who felt high presence in response to an avatar being more likely to eat unhealthy food, whereas women who felt high presence were more likely not to eat candy.

Taken as a whole, the reviewed research streams and findings in the area of VR and presence have interesting implications. First, they show the diversity of topics in health that may be addressed using VR. Second, they point to the importance of considering presence (chiefly spatial presence and self presence) in this research as a measure of technological effectiveness. Third, they show the potential of VR as a tool for creating high levels of presence with equally strong impacts on healthcare outcomes. For IDSS, the work on VR and presence for health suggests that creating high presence-inducing VR experiences can make users feel more in virtual spaces and connected to avatars, potentially making them more motivated to use the systems and also increasing the ability to do so. Research on these connections can help identify the extent to which VR applications for IDSS create presence leading to further outcomes of interest.

4.2 Health Research on Agents/Other Technologies and Presence

Agents have been the focus of a handful of presence and health investigations to date. David, Cai, Lu, and Jeong [13] looked at the effects of gender on responses to an anthropomorphic computer help agent. Specifically, they were interested in how the match (or mismatch) between agent gender and respondent gender affected social presence dimensions and other outcomes. They found that agent gender did not have a strong effect on males, but for females a female agent was rated significantly higher on co-presence, attention, and understanding. The female agent was also rated higher by females than an interface without agent cues. This suggests that agent design and corresponding social presence can have an effect on healthcare, by affecting outcomes such as attention to and understanding of health messages.

Huang [18] examined how the interactivity and expressiveness of agents impacted dimensions of social presence along with memory, attitude, and behavioral intention toward a health message focused on drunk driving. Findings were mixed, with both expressiveness and interactivity impacting presence dimensions. Interactivity of an agent also impacted learning, though expressiveness did not. Attitude change and behavioral intention were not affected by either manipulation, contrary to expectations.

In a similar study that attempted to better explain variable relationships using theory, Skalski and Tamborini [33] investigated the social presence and persuasion effects of a health interactive social agent, using information processing theory as a guide. They predicted that an interactive social agent (versus one that passively communicated information) would cause users to experience more social presence. Social presence was then expected to compel listeners to process health information more centrally, leading to a more positive attitude and behavioral intention toward a health issue (blood pressure checkups). Findings were generally in line with expectations, showing the potential of computer agents to serve as effective communicators of health information.

Additional studies, focused on technologies other than agents, provide further insight into the relationship between presence and health outcomes. Hawkins et al. [17] explored how interactivity relates to social presence, in response to a variety of interventions directed toward breast cancer patients. They found that an Internet-based system scored low on both interactivity and social presence, while a system involving a human "Cancer Mentor" scored the highest. This highlights deficiencies in current technologies, though these should diminish over time as the technologies improve. Alem, Hansen, and Li [2] tested a telemedicine system that allows a specialist at a major hospital to direct teams in smaller, remote hospitals. Their findings indicated that, while individual differences played a role in clinician presence, there may still be a relationship between presence and outcomes such as ease of technology use and satisfaction with video quality. Bouchard, Robillard, Marchand, Renaud, and Riva [7] investigated how closely patients and therapists bond during videoconferencing sessions. They found that presence related positively to bond strength, suggesting the concept's importance in telepsychotherapy. Sponselee, de Kort, and Meijnders [35] found mixed results however when testing the role of presence in relieving stress through mediated restorative environments.

As a final note, Sundar, Oeldorf-Hirsch, and Garga [37] advance an intriguing overall framework for exploring and explaining connections between technology and presence, known as the MAIN model. It suggests that affordances of technology (i.e., Modality, Agency, Interactivity, and Navigability) transmit cues that trigger cognitive heuristics leading to presence. This model sheds further light on how technologies such as IDSS may induce presence. For example, if they have agency, the agency can trigger the *social presence heuristic*, which says "I can sense the other, therefore I am present with him/her" [37, p. 225]. The navigability of the system can create another *browsing heuristic* that further facilitates presence through exploration. The research reviewed in this section on agents and other healthcare technology applications suggests that they have an impact on presence (specifically social presence in the case of agents), and that this presence can be increased through affordances such as interactivity. Moreover, the findings once again show how presence has a positive impact on health communication outcomes, further cementing the concept's importance to achieving them.

5 Conclusion and Recommendations

The experience of presence is a complex process depending on the interaction of media form, content, and user characteristics. Nevertheless, it holds tremendous value as a tool for understanding IDSS and other healthcare technologies. The advantage of considering the human, psychological side of technology use (i.e., presence) over just hardware or technologies themselves is that presence is a common, measurable outcome of *any* media experience, with predictable results. Instead of having to account for the potentially limitless number of features that might differentiate current and future technologies along qualitative dimensions, focusing on presence allows researchers to concentrate on a single enduring aspect of human experience that varies along a continuum. Presence measures can be used to experimentally compare across different manipulations of media form and content, such as options for IDSS, to determine which combinations lead users to perceive the most "naturalness" or "realness." In that sense, presence functions as a "manipulation check" for technological effectiveness, expected to relate positively to dependent variables of interest.

Presence also functions as an organizing concept for research on new technologies like VR and agents. It has been studied by scholars in diverse fields, including engineering, computer science, communication, media studies, and psychology. Theory and research on presence helps unite these traditions as they work toward common goals, such as understanding the distinctions between real and mediated experiences and manufacturing mediated experiences that seem real. Important issues like these cannot be fully addressed simply by testing relationships between technologies and outcomes. For example, it may be that certain types of IDSS are more effective, but why? Answering this question requires the inclusion of mediating variables such as presence in research, which are necessary for the construction of explanatory models. Models, in turn, help build theory and accomplish the goals of science, i.e., description, explanation, and prediction [16]. Explanation makes prediction easier by pinpointing variables that can cause a particular outcome (e.g., presence). Given the obvious value in predicting outcomes such as how to more effectively deliver healthcare information, explanation and prediction should be considered in tandem. Following are some additional recommendations concerning presence and IDSS for healthcare:

- *Consider presence dimensions separately and only focus on relevant ones*: There are many types and sub-dimensions of presence that have been advanced over the years. Although some researchers have indexed these to create an overall measure of presence, separate dimensions of the concept should be treated separately, as recommended by Bracken and Skalski [10]. One reason for this is that the types may not relate the same to independent and dependent variables of interest in a study because their conceptual meanings are different. This is especially true for spatial presence, social presence, and self presence, which represent distinct experiences. IDSS through VR technology would probably affect a user's spatial presence or self presence, whereas IDSS agents would probably affect a user's sense of social presence. The choice of presence type should depend on the type of technology being investigated and other variables of interest. And when in doubt, it is fine to consider multiple types of presence, provided that they are treated separate from one another.

- *Measure presence using established methods*: Presence measurement has been a major subject of inquiry for scholars studying the concept, resulting in the development of many validated scales and other suggestions for measurement [e.g., 21, 22]. These measurement tools are freely available, for the most part, and their use is encouraged. They not only remove the hardships involved in developing new measures but also allow for easy cross-study comparisons.

- *Draw upon the large accumulated body of presence literature when needed*: In the short history of presence scholarship, an impressive body of knowledge has accumulated. Lombard and Jones [27] identified more than 1,400 articles addressing the concept. These range from the very technical articles typically appearing in the journal *Presence: Teleoperators and Virtual Environments* to conceptual pieces appearing in journals such as *Communication Theory*. Research findings on presence provide a useful springboard for determining, for example, technology form and content variables that can maximize presence. The presence literature can therefore suggest ideal designs for new IDSS or ways to make existing ones more effective.

- *Remember the advantages of VR and agents as "superhuman" technologies*: As shown in the work of Jeremy Bailenson and colleagues, VR can not only be used to simulate real life but also to surpass it. Students training to be heart surgeons, for example, might benefit from a simulator that allows them to operate on a virtual heart with a specific problem, to learn how to repair it without risk to a patient. Such a simulator might also allow the user to instantly change to another type of problem, or even another organ, making VR superior in some ways to other forms of education. Computer agents, likewise, far exceed a human's capacity for information storage and retrieval. They can surpass any medical professional in information sharing. These systems are therefore of tremendous value as healthcare tools, especially if they are designed with presence in mind and users can interact with them in natural, lifelike fashion.

- *Conduct research on how IDSS technologies and variables relate to presence*: A final and important step is to conduct research to empirically establish the connection between presence and IDSS technologies and variables. Power [29] traces the development of decision support systems (DSS) and identifies a number of historical types, including model driven DSS, data driven DSS, communications DSS, document DSS, knowledge-driven DSS, and Web-based DSS. Research on Communication and Web-based DSS are obvious linkage points between the media-focused presence literature and the IDSS literature. In addition, IDSS scholarship calls attention to the importance of variables such as artificial intelligence, which may also impact presence in the manner discussed earlier. Understanding how healthcare technology applications affect presence can be valuable for physicians and patients alike. Early research on computer-based clinical decision support systems, for example, revealed that the systems have been useful in some areas, such as drug dosing and preventive care, but lacking in others, such as diagnosis [19]. The inability of certain technologies to induce presence may have played a role in these outcomes; accounting for presence may help improve their effectiveness.

In addition to giving an overview of the concept of the presence and its causes, this chapter demonstrates the benefits of considering presence in health research using advanced technologies such as VR and agents. It also suggests areas for further inquiry by IDSS scholars. It is relatively easy to add presence measures to IDSS studies, and doing so can reveal much about users' psychological reactions to intelligent decision support systems for healthcare. As Lombard and Ditton [26] suggest, presence is central to our understanding of the relationship between people and technology, "at the heart of it all."

References

1. Alcaniz, M., Banos, R., Botella, C., Rey, B.: The EMMA Project: Emotions as a determinant of presence. PsychNology 1(2), 141–150 (2003)
2. Alem, L., Hansen, S., Li, J.: Evaluating clinicians' experience in a telemedicine application: A presence perspective. In: Proc. OZCHI 2006 Conf., pp. 46–54. ACM Press, NY (2006)
3. Bailenson, J., Patel, K., Nielsen, A., Bajscy, R., Jung, S., Kurillo, G.: The effect of interactivity on learning physical actions in virtual reality. Media Psychology 11(3), 354–376 (2008)
4. Biocca, F., Delaney, B.: Immersive virtual reality technology. In: Biocca, F., Levy, M. (eds.) Communication in the age of virtual reality. Lawrence Erlbaum Associates, Hillsdale (1995)
5. Biocca, F., Harms, C., Burgoon, J.K.: Toward a more robust theory and measure of social presence: Review and suggested criteria. Presence: Teleoperators and Virtual Environments 12(5), 456–480 (2003)
6. Biocca, F., Levy, M.: Communication in the age of virtual reality. Lawrence Erlbaum Associates, Hillsdale (1995)

7. Bouchard, S., Robillard, G., Marchand, A., Renaud, P., Riva, G.: Presence and the bond between patients and their psychotherapists in the cognitive-behavior therapy of panic disorder with agoraphobia delivered in videoconference. In: Proceedings of the 10th Annual International Workshop on Presence, Barcelona, pp. 25–27 (2007)
8. Bracken, C.C.: Presence and image quality: The case of high definition television. Media Psychology 7(2), 191–205 (2005)
9. Bracken, C.C., Botta, R.: Telepresence and television. In: Bracken, C.C., Skalski, P. (eds.) Immersed in media: Telepresence in everyday life, pp. 39–62. Routledge, New York (2010)
10. Bracken, C.C., Skalski, P.: Immersed in media: Telepresence in everyday life. Routledge, New York (2010)
11. Brown, S., Nunez, D., Blake, E.H.: Using virtual reality to provide nutritional support to HIV+ women. In: Proceedings of the 8th Annual International Workshop on Presence, London (2005)
12. Castelnuovo, G., Lo Priore, D., Di, L., Gaggioli, A., Riva, G., Da, L.: The sense of presence in a sample of patients with neuropsychological dysfunctions during a VR enhanced cognitive rehabilitation. In: Proceedings of the 6th annual international workshop on presence, Aalborg (2003)
13. David, P., Cai, L., Lu, T., Jeong, I.: Gender identification with an anthropomorphic computer agent: A social presence approach. In: Proceedings of the 6th annual international workshop on presence, Aalborg (2003)
14. Fox, J., Bailenson, J.: Virtual self-modeling: The effects of vicarious reinforcement and identification on exercise behaviors. Media Psychology 12(1), 1–25 (2009)
15. Fox, J., Bailenson, J.: Virtual experiences, physical behaviors: The effect of presence on imitation of an eating avatar. Paper presented at the 59th annual conference of the International Communication Association, Chicago, IL (2009)
16. Hanna, J.F.: Explanation, prediction, description, and information theory. Synthese 20, 308–334 (1969)
17. Hawkins, R., Han, J., Pingree, S., Baker, T., Roberts, L., Shaw, B.: Interactivity and presence of three eHealth interventions. Paper presented at the 57th annual conference of the International Communication Association, San Francisco, CA,
18. Huang, H.: Effects of interactivity and expressiveness on perceived social presence, memory and persuasion in interactive health communications. In: Proceedings of the 6th annual international workshop on presence, Aalborg (2003)
19. Hunt, D.L., Haynes, R.B., Hanna, S.E., Smith, K.: Effects of computer based clinical decision support systems on physician performance and patient outcomes: A systematic review. Journal of the American Medical Association 280, 1339–1346 (1998)
20. ISPR (International Society for Presence Research) (2000) The concept of presence: Explication statement, `http://ispr.info/` (retrieved June 20, 2009)
21. Insko, B.E.: Measuring presence: Subjective, behavioral, and physiological methods. In: Riva, G., Davide, F., IJsselsteijn, W.A. (eds.) Being there: Concepts, effects and measurement of user presence in synthetic environments. IOS Press, Amsterdam (2003)
22. International Society for Presence Research (n.d.) Tools to measure presence, `http://www.temple.edu/ispr/frame_measure.htm` (retrieved May 15, 2009)
23. Lee, K.M.: Presence, explicated. Communication Theory 14(1), 27–50 (2004)

24. Lombard, M.: The promise and peril of telepresence. In: Bracken, C.C., Skalski, P. (eds.) Immersed in media: Telepresence in everyday life, pp. 197–228. Routledge, New York (2010)
25. Lombard, M.: Direct responses to people on the screen: Television and personal space. Communication Research 22(3), 288–324 (1995)
26. Lombard, M., Ditton, T.: At the heart of it all: The concept of presence. Journal of Computer Mediated Communication 3(2) (1997) `http://jcmc.indiana.edu/vol3/issue2/lombard.html` (retrieved May 1, 2010)
27. Lombard, M., Jones, M.: Identifying the (tele)presence literature. PsychNology Journal 5(2), 197–206 (2007)
28. Neuendorf, K.A., Lieberman, E.: Film: The original immersive medium. In: Bracken, C.C., Skalski, P. (eds.) Immersed in media: Telepresence in everyday life, pp. 9–38. Routledge, New York (2010)
29. Power, D.J.: A brief history of decision support systems4.0. DSSResources.COM (2007), `http://DSSResources.COM/history/dsshistory.html` (retrieved April 20, 2010)
30. Reeves, B.R.: Being there: Television as symbolic versus natural experience. Stanford University, Institute for Communication Research, Stanford, CA (1991) (unpublished manuscript)
31. Reeves, B., Nass, C.: The media equation: How people treat computers, television and new media like real people and places. Cambridge University Press, Cambridge (1996)
32. Sheridan, T.B.: Musings on telepresence and virtual presence. Presence: Teleoperators and Virtual Environments 1(1), 120–126 (1992)
33. Skalski, P., Tamborini, R.: The role of social presence in interactive agent-based persuasion. Media Psychology 10(3), 385–413 (2007)
34. Skalski, P., Tamborini, R., Shelton, A., Buncher, M., Lindmark, P.: Mapping the road to fun: Natural video game controllers, presence, and game enjoyment. New Media & Society (in press) (forthcoming)
35. Sponselee, A.M., Kort, Y.A.W., de Meijnders, A.L.: Healing media: The moderating role of presence in restoring from stress in a mediated environment. In: Alcaniz Raya, M., Rey Solaz, B. (eds.) PRESENCE 2004: Proceedings of the 7th Annual International Workshop on Presence Valencia, Spain, pp. 197–203 (2004)
36. Steuer, J.: Defining virtual reality: Dimensions determining telepresence. Journal of Communication 42(4), 73–93 (1992)
37. Sundar, S.S., Oeldorf-Hirsch, A., Garga, A.: A cognitive-heuristics approach to understanding presence in virtual environments. In: Spagnolli, A., Gamberini, L. (eds.) PRESENCE 2008: Proceedings of the 11th Annual International Workshop on Presence, Padova, Italy, pp. 219–228 (2008)
38. Turban, E., Aronson, J., Liang, T.: Decision support systems and intelligent systems. Prentice Hall, Englewood Cliffs (2004)
39. Whitbred, R., Skalski, P., Bracken, C.C., Lieberman, E.: When richer is poorer: Understanding the influence of channel richness and presence on the introduction of a mission statement. PsychNology 8(1), 115–139 (2010)
40. Witmer, B.G., Singer, M.J.: Measuring presence in virtual environments: A presence questionnaire. Presence 7, 225–240 (1998)
41. Wirth, W., Hartmann, T., Boecking, S., Vorderer, P., Klimmt, C., Schramm, H., et al.: A process model of the formation of spatial presence experiences. Media Psychology 9, 493–525 (2007)

Chapter 11
Witnessed Presence in Merging Realities in Healthcare Environments

Caroline Nevejan and Frances Brazier

Dynamic Adaptive Systems Design - Faculty Technology, Policy and Management
Delft Technical University, the Netherlands
nevejan@xs4all.nl, F.M.Brazier@tudelft.nl

Abstract. Witnessing is core to the design of social interaction. This chapter explores the role of witnessing from different perspectives. The first perspective focuses on witnessing in its social and psychological consequences. Response-ability, address- ability, the performance of testimony and transparency of subject position determine how individuals perceive/witness each other. The second perspective focuses on the impact of technology on witnessing and introduces the YUTPA framework as a tool for the design and orchestration of witnessing in technology environments. The third, fourth and fifth sections discuss initial results of exploratory research performed in the Netherlands and in India. This research shows that the way in which witnessing is orchestrated affects the psychological well-being of the people involved: it can be beneficial or detrimental. These results demonstrate the need to explicitly design witnessing along the four dimensions of the YUTPA model: space, time, action and relation. The sixth section addresses a third perspective, the technological perspective that focuses on the design of large scale socio-technological systems. The conclusion of this chapter argues that health systems that affect the psychological well being of the people involved must both be designed to take witnessing into account but also to be used appropriately.

Keywords: Witness, Technology, Presence, Healthcare, Cyber Therapy, Systems Design, Time, Place, Action, Relation, Trust, Collaboration, Socio-Technological systems.

1 Introduction

Today's virtual environments for healthcare, eg those created for cyber therapy and behavioural training, orchestrate social interaction. The real world and virtual world are often intentionally blurred through the use of technology. Therapist(s) and client(s) witness each other directly or indirectly by way of technology. The choice of technology and options for communication determines how people interact, how people perceive each other, how they can be witness to each other, and how they can take responsibility for each other and themselves.

In most of these systems, information about clients is only accessible to the therapists. The introduction of the Electronic Patient Files (EPD) in 2008,

S. Brahnam & L.C. Jain (Eds.): Adv. Comput. Intell. Paradigms in Healthcare 5, SCI 326, pp. 201–227.
springerlink.com

approved by the Dutch Parliament in 2008, has changed the situation drastically. Each and every citizen in the Netherlands has an EPD, unless he/she formally refuses. The ambition of the EPD is to provide complete documentation on each patient instantaneously at any place of care, with explicit patient permission. This documentation, large repositories of medical, psychological and health knowledge, may be tailored to personal needs, giving advice, support or warn people in specific situations. Data-mining programs, software agents, and small bots can easily become medical friends, coaches and even therapists. These friends interact with the 'data-identity' of human beings. The data-identity acquires more and more agency over time. As the number of specific virtual environments for changing human behaviour is increasing fast and the development of larger healthcare systems progresses, the new interaction between human beings and systems demands rigorous analysis. Note that large databases also make it possible to create new kinds of interaction between the healthcare system, the insurance companies, employers and individual human beings.

This chapter focuses on how well-being of human beings in technology environments can be orchestrated. It argues that the design of witnessing is crucial and shows that in each of the four dimensions of the YUTPA framework (time, place, action, relation) specific issues for the design of witnessing in larger social technical systems can be identified. YUTPA is the acronym for 'being with You in Unity of Time, Place and Action".

Section 2 introduces an interdisciplinary social science and philosophical perspective on witnessing after which the YUTPA framework for design and analysis is shortly explained. Section 3, 4 and 5 present current exploratory research in which the YUTPA framework is used to better understand possibilities for witnessing in a variety of presence designs. Section 6 takes the results of the exploratory study and formulates possible implications for system design. The discussion in Section 7 relates insights and concepts to healthcare as a context for design.

2 Witnessing and the YUTPA Framework

The performance of presence and the enactment of being, presuppose the presence of other beings and as a result witnessed presence. Before language is uttered, human beings recognize spatiotemporal trajectories of other beings setting the parameters for any sequential interaction [1]. Witnessing can be distinguished from observing, in which cognition plays a significant role, and from perceiving, in which sensorial input has dominance. Witnessing, as proposed in this chapter, builds upon perception and observation but also includes the possibility to act upon what is witnessed. Being witness includes taking of responsibility by acting upon, or testifying about, the perception and observation of the situation to which a person is witness. Witnessed presence, operates on all levels of consciousness: it is one of the building blocks of social rules, defined by space and time. Social rules determine the social structures that human beings construct [2].

In Law, in communities, in businesses and organizations the persona of the witness is distinct. In most judicial systems the witness has to be sworn in. By doing so the witness accepts responsibility to speak the truth. In other words, being witness involves accepting responsibility for what happens next. When being witnessed, any act becomes a deed [3]. Perception and observation involve judgement on several levels of consciousness. Witnessing refers to the fact that the persona of the witness embodies the possibility to act upon and/or to testify about the act. When witnessed, the perception or observation of an act is considered from the perspective of possible re-action and contextualizes perception and observation in the strive for well-being and survival in which the essence of presence is to be found [4]. Vice versa, when human beings feel there is no possibility to act (or re-act), people detach themselves from a situation and take a moral distance others, their actions and even to their own self [5].

In traditional social structures witnessing assumes a sharing of time and place, being in relation to each other, and having the possibility to act within the interaction that is taking place. In new space and time configurations facilitated by technology, such relations are not as easily acquired. Millions of people, however, use these technologies to sustain personal and professional relationships. A variety of presence designs have emerged and in all of these presence designs people find ways to communicate, to develop relationships between people in series of interactions. Having a conversation, making a phone call, sending an email, postings on the Internet and the variety of possibilities to chat or Skype are all specific presence designs, which contribute in a series of social interactions to the building up or breaking down of trust [3]. To have presence requires agency; to be able to perform presence; to be able to 'enact' being [6]. The way in which people are witness to each other, in the variety of presence designs, influences how trust is built [7].

Human kind has developed a variety of social structures in which witnessing is distinct: family structures, community structures, organizational structures, business structures, judicial structures, learning structures, national and transnational structures. In all of these structures people are witness to each other. This deeply influences how people interact. Conflict and tension are a given, but the way in which people handle conflict and tensions in one social structure differs from another. In a large comparative studyFukuyama finds that 'high trust' societies are beneficial for human beings: people are happier and live longer [8]. Business theory argues that high trust in organizations creates more success [9]. Stephenson describes trust as the sort of glue that holds social structures together [10]. In the establishment of trust, witnessing plays a significant role [7].

Oliver claims that the capability of witnessing - to witness, to bear witness and to be in dialogue with one's inner witness - is fundamental to being human [11]. She argues that being witness is characterized by the possibility of response-ability and address-ability. Response-ability refers to the subjectivity, which allows a person to respond to the person who testifies. Oliver connects this to ethical responsibility.[1] Address-ability refers to the being able to address one's testimony to another human being who will listen. Response-ability and address-ability function in relation with the 'inner witness' every human being has. Oliver argues that

[1] This resonates with Damasio's suggestion that in the strive for well-being and survival, also the ethical ground is to be found [5]. To hurt others makes one's own environment unsafe.

when being victimized or having to deal with trauma, people need to restore the dialogue with their inner witness. Only through the performance of testimony in which one can address a person who is willing to be witness and therefore is willing to respond and share responsibility for the performance of testimony, a person can transform traumatic experiences in such a way that repetition will stop. The joint responsibility of witnessing, as a source for the re-emerging truth, is needed to be able to give testimony of traumatic experiences of oppression and victimization, argues Oliver. The psychological process that happens as a result of giving testimony, in which the unsaid can be communicated, is transformation. Such transformation processes are part of all stages of life, of being mother and child, falling in love, developing friendships and more. However, 'false witnessing' has to be addressed in this context, Oliver concludes that if a person is not in the proper subject position witnessing cannot be. A subject position is defined by the social structures in which an individual acts and therefore has knowledge about. One has to be a farmer to give testimony about farming for example and not an actress. Subject positionneeds to be made transparent for witnessed presence to be significant. Oliver argues convincingly that through witnessing and being witnessed and through the dialogue of one's inner witness, the essence of human presence develops [11].

The presence design of Oliver's work on witnessing, assumes a sharing of time and place, being in relation to each other and having the possibility to act within the interaction that is taking place. Current technologies challenge this presence design by providing new possibilities to transcend time and place at a high speed and large scale. Presence, as such, has never been a given, argues IJsselsteijn, it is a trade-off [12]. At a certain moment in a certain place, given the specific context and perceived sensorial input, a certain status quo is accepted. The way sensorial input is understood is a trade-off. Eyes for example can only handle a limited amount of input in distance, colours and more. In day-to-day social presences human beings make trade-offs all the time. When a woman meets a big man in a dark alley at night there may be a moment that she decides to run without having to know exactly how strong the guy is or where he is from.

Also the way people adapt to new technologies is determined by making trade-offs [12]. When film was introduced more than a century ago, an audience would scream and shiver when a train wouldhead their direction on screen. Through collective experience the understanding of the train on screen changed and 'screen-reality' has been accepted in its own right as part of day-to-day reality. These adaptation processes are time-based and are specific for certain periods in time in certain cultures and for certain generations as well [13]. Media technologies such as television, mobile phones, videogames, Internet and also the use of large databases and visualization of data-sets in professional environments for example, all cause new trade-offs to emerge.

The fact that presence is a trade-off, creates the possibility to design this trade-off. Not only time and place have a distinct influence how the trade-off is made, but also the relation between people and the possibility to act, The trade-off of presence determines how witnessing contributes to the ability to build or destroy trust [7]. The YUTPA framework has been developed to analyze trade-offs in presence design [3]. YUTPA is the acronym for "being with You in Unity of Time, Place and Action". In the YUTPA framework each specific presence design is analyzed along 4 dimensions: time, place, action, relation. Sharing time and place and being in a sustainable relationship with each other upon which one is allowed to act, is the ultimate YUTPA configuration in which trust increases or diminishes and in which 'true witnessing', in Oliver's terms, may happen [11].

The 4 dimensions between Now and not-Now, Here and not-Here, You and not-You, Do and not-Do,influence the ability to build a sustainable relationship as defined by trust. Not sharing place, not sharing time, not being in relation and not having any possibility to act creates zero dynamics for building or breaking down trust. When not sharing time and place with someone with whom one is deeply related, trust travels easily and technology mediates this trust. When making a YUTPA analysis, a rigorous describing of each of the four dimensions in relation to the other three sheds light on how the trade-off in a specific presence design is made.

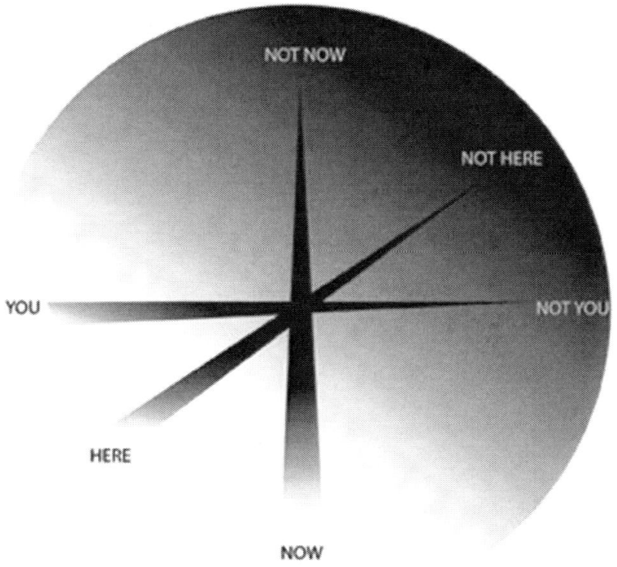

Fig. 1. The YUTPA framework defines in four dimensions the relation between presence and a sustainable relationship defined by trust. The black and white parts of the sphere present the possibility to act (Do/notDo).

3 Exploring Witnessed Presence and Systems Engineering

To explore the different ways in which witnessing has emerged in new forms of interaction between man and machineNevejan and Brazier (authors of this chapter) designed the qualitative studythat is presented in this section. Initial results will be shared in section 4 and 5. To explore Witnessed Presence artists, designers, engineers and business developers, whose day-to-day practice is deeply affected by technology have been interviewed by Nevejan. The choice of experts is not arbitrary. They have been chosen on the basis of their reputation, knowledge and experience. The intention of the interviews is to make their tacit knowledge on witnessed presence surface,to discover words and concepts related to witnessed presence and its four dimensions. The first results of this study provide a rational and ethical basis upon which applications and infrastructures for healthcare can be analyzed and designed.

3.1 Methodology

To explore 'witnessed presence' 17 interviews have been conducted with designers, social scientists, engineers, artists and business developers in the Netherlands and in India. The people interviewed are fluent in more than one professional language and have a rich experience on which their knowledge, insights and skills are based. All of the experts have an established reputation in their field. The interviews can be considered as acts of Parrèsia[2], the ancient Greek concept for knowledge that evolves from personal and professional experience in respected contexts [14].

---

[2] The Greeks made a distinction between Epistème and Parrèsia. Epistème refers to knowledge production in which objective knowledge is produced by logical reasoning and by providing evidence. Modern science is largely based on this tradition. Parrèsia refers to the act of speaking the truth from a specific personal experience and a recognized ethical position. Parrèsia is not easily accepted as a method for producing knowledge in the scientific realm. Yet in contrast to this, in the professional realm a personal speaking of the truth that derives its authority from experience and a recognized ethical position is widely accepted and appreciated. According to the Greeks, to be able to speak the truth a person needs to have the right attitude. "In Parrèsia, the speaker uses his freedom and chooses frankness instead of persuasion, truth instead of falsehood or silence, the risk of death instead of life and security, criticism instead of flattery, and moral duty instead of self–interest and moral apathy" [14]. The process of revealing truth to oneself involves formulating, taking distance, evaluating, analyzing and re–formulating. Foucault was inspired on Parrèsia as a methodology for analysis by Plutarch: "These exercises are part of what we could call an "aesthetics of the self". For one does not have to take up a position or role towards oneself as that of a judge pronouncing a verdict. One can comport oneself towards oneself in the role of a technician, of a craftsman, of an artist, who — from time to time — stops working, examines what he is doing, reminds himself of the rules of his art, and compares these rules with what he has achieved thus far." [14].

The interviews have a very open character taking the experience and expertise of the experts as perspective. The interviews can be best characterized as structured conversations in which current thinking is shared and explored in the different discourses and disciplines in which the interviewed people work. The interviewer's role can be characterized as being witness to a performance of testimony on the interviewed person's professional experience and reflection on this experience; offering address-ability and taking response-ability in a context in which subject positions are clear. The interviewer knew the subjects professionally. In all of the interviews the notion of witnessed presence and the four dimensions of the YUTPA framework are addressed in relation to the practice and insights of the expert interviewed.

Fundamental in this study is its interdisciplinary nature. The specific understanding of a phenomenon and the words that describe a phenomenon in relation to other concepts and phenomena in a specific discipline, are diverse and cannot be easily transposed to other disciplines. The understanding of interdisciplinary research in this study builds upon the awareness that such research requires multilingual skills as well as an open attitude [15]. Specific requirements have been met to facilitate the interdisciplinary nature of this study. In the first place the research question offers a perspective to which the different disciplines can relate. Secondly the research context provides a climate ofexperience with interdisciplinary research in which a manner of conversation has been developed in which terms and concepts are under constant exploration. Thirdly, both investigators have acquired multi lingual capacity in many interdisciplinary projects before. Last, but not least, all of the people interviewed have shown to be willing to endure the uncomfortability that is part of exploring new territories. This interdisciplinary exploratory research project is not a comparative study. Through the accumulation of insights from different domains and practices, a sketch of witnessing in technology environments is made.

In the interviews the perspective of the actor in an agent-actor environment is central. This is also the focus in the presentation of the results. The research informs experiments in the field of collaborative distributed work, the modelling of systems for crisis management and inspires further thinking on the ethics and implications of system foundations.

To offer maximum transparency and increase the validity of this study all interviews have been filmed and the source material has been published on the Internet. Each interview lasts one hour, filmed in the presence of a camera and a cameraman.

The interviews have been filmed with a wide angle to provide an impression of the way people move and gesticulate while being deeply involved in expressing their views. The complete transcript of the individual interviews including film fragments can be accessed at http://www.systemsdesign.tbm.tudelft.nl/witness. Note that in this chapter references refer to the opinions expressed in the interviews themselves, often introducing the expert briefly.

4 Results: Exploring the Context of Witnessed Presence and Systems Engineering

The nature of the interaction between human beings and systems influences the way presence is witnessed. This section first focuses (1) on interaction with technology, (2) on how biological, social and algorithmic realities merge and (3) on how partial perspectives change through transaction.

4.1 Interacting with Technology

For many centuries being witness referred to an 'inscribing with the body' one's presence and therefore being able to testify, as formulated by new media artist Hazra [16]. Physically presence was needed to be witness to a situation. Today's technologies, with their different scale and speed of collecting and distributing data, offer a perspective that human kind has not been able to perceive before. People can be witness to situations thousands of miles away. Both on the micro level as happens for example in molecular science as well as on the macro level with technologies like satellite, database technologies and the Internet, human beings can perceive realities they could not perceive before. As users of technology human beings become actors in these environments. Both technology and human beings are in a process of change because they interact.

In traditional communities of artisans witnessed presence is fundamental, argues designer Panghaal [17]. In addition to working with companies such as Nokia and Motorala, Panghaal also works with communities of craftspeople who for example work with steel in the same way as people would do 2000 years ago. Artisans do not make things in the past or project their work in the future but create now and here, Panghaal explains. It is physical work and if the body is not centredthe artisan will not be capable to do the work the next day. The interaction between body and material is profound. The material actually changes the human being who works with it. Like material, also the interaction between technology and human being affects people profoundly. Panghaal cites the example of the mobile phone, which has a side effect of not having to make decisions anymore about being at a certain place at a certain time to be able to meet [17].

The interviews support the assumption that technology has impact on the four dimensions of the YUTPA framework by changing e.g. scale, speed, perspective, granularity, and rhythm. Technology, however, also communicates concepts of ethics and aesthetics at the same time. Van Splunter, computer scientist, makes a convincing argument that when making a chair a concept of sitting is communicated, when making an email program a concept of communication is created and so on [18].In architecture, where technology has a great impact on the tools and materials that can be used, algorithmic reality offers a new sense of aesthetics for which people can be sensitive. A new visual logic is emerging, according to architect Jansma, even though visual logic cannot be expressed in language as such [19]. Technology affects human perception and action and while doing so it communicates concepts of ethics and aesthetics at the same time as well.

4.2 Biological, Social and Algorithmic Realities Merge

Infrastructures and people adapt and this is part of the evolutionary process of social technical systems in which people live, argues anthropologist and designer Sood [20]. However, argues Sood, people know what they deal with. Even when dealing with complex technological systems or robots or agents, human beings will recognize in a limited amount of time whether they deal with something human or technological.

Today's technology, however, offers limited sensorial experiences of quality by itself and therefore it mostly depends on references of profound experiences in other realms of life argues Panghaal [17]. Interfaces are designed to give a sense of gravity or force feedback, specific personalization is made possible and lower layers of technology are hidden. Differences between biological, social and technological input are often purposefully blurred to provide a frame of reference, to support acceptance, making it difficult for users to distinguish the roles, argue computer scientists Warnier [21] and Quillinan [22].

Not only biological and social reality define people's sense of the world around the globe, also technological reality has deeply invaded human beings perception of self, illustrates Hazra[16]. Medical technology and information and communication technology merge with social and biological perception into one image of the human body and its environment in common practices of all sorts. Taking the example of sleep,Hazra explains that a person has the sense of sleep, he or she may use a monitor to be aware of personal patterns of sleep and there are statistics on patterns of sleep. In the experience of paying attention to sleep all of these kinds of information about the self merge into one feeling and knowledge base about sleep. Because different realities merge, a variety of presences may exist and technology is capable of offering new perspectives on the self from a 'third point' as Hazra calls it [16].

4.3 Partial Personal Perspective Changes through Transaction

In the merging realities it is important to realize that each individual person makes his or her own specific configuration of different realities according to personal need. When sleep is not an issue, only the biological reality may be a reference for a person. Only when sleep becomes problematic do other realities merge. In health situations personal reality configurations are distinct between different people. The merging of biological and social reality, as in the nature-nurture debate, already creates lots of fundamental confusion. The variety of presences technology facilitates, and the large information and communication repositories it produces, makes the confusion even more profound. The fact that realities merge does not imply that human beings perceive more of what happens or perceive in a more profound way. Merging realities influence individuals' mental maps and understanding of the personal body and of the contexts in which people find themselves. But also in larger merging realities human beings have partial perspectives. Presence is a universal concept and witnessing is not, according to communications scholar Parthasarathi [23].

Bawa, scholar on politics of land, finds that even the way people understand 'the land' has become a complex issue in which different realities merge. Ownership, political and social relations, business, maps, television and databases define how people perceive their urban environment. Real and virtual flows merge but she finds that in the merging realities, the social-political position of human beings remains to be distinct when being witness to what happens [24]. In her work on religious contexts, on housing politics and in the warzone of Srinadar, she finds that without being in dialogue there is no interaction and the being witness to each other becomes a mere judging [24]. Parthasarathi argues from a different realm that the social-political position of people defines what they can be witness to even when different realities have merged. If one is not in dialogue or in transaction with a specific situation, one cannot be witness to that situation [23].[3] From yet another perspective Wilson, technical director of an online software company, supports this argument as well [25]. For her, the different realities of the online and offline world merge in her personal life, but do not merge at all in her social life. Because most of her friends do not know her online life, she cannot share this world and they cannot be witness to a large part of her life. There is no language in which she can express this other world to people who are not part of it [25].

A partial perspective can only be changed by transaction, argues Parthasarathi [23]. Only when being in transaction can one be witness to each other and perceive new parts of the merging realities through these transactions. Social political positions, in the merging biological, social and algorithmic realities, define with whom and with what one can be in transaction with. In healthcare other perspectives are mostly created when being confronted with implications of illness or pathological patterns of behaviour. Also here, the need to develop other partial perspectives only evolves when having to enter into new transactions in order to safeguard well-being and life. Hazra argues that the realization of merging realities demands for a new ethics of responsibility, which is no longer based in presence alone [16]. Especially for healthcare such an ethic has to be explored.

5 Results: Exploring Witnessing in the Four Dimensions of the YUTPA Framework in Relation to Future Healthcare Issues

Time, place, relation and the possibility to act define the subject position of a human being in the social structures he or she is engaged with. When discussing the construction of time, place, action and relation between human beings and systems it is necessary to make a distinction between two kinds of interaction. There are interactions in which a human being directly interacts with the system and there are interactions in which technology mediates human interaction. In healthcare both interactions take place separately and intertwined in certain cases. This

[3] In an analysis of the media-coverage of the Mumbai attacks, he argues that because the reporters were all familiar with the hotels that were bombed, the media coverage focused on these hotels. The railway station, where many more people died, was hardly mentioned because the reporters, nor the owners of the television stations, were regular users of the railway station. To them the railway station had no significance.

distinction is made in the following four sections on the dimensions: time, place, action and relation.

5.1 Time Is the Beholder of Trust in Online Collaboration

When designing processes, systems and applications, time is one of the features to be constructed: rhythm, instances of synchronization or random noise. Design of time is one of the four dimensions that is distinct in the experience of the users of a system.

Human beings and systems have very different structures in time. Human beings breathe, have heartbeats, get tired.They need to sleep, drink and eat. Human beings live only for a limited amount of time and go though life cycles. A human being's memory is distinct, specific events are remembered and others are not, whole chunks of time, disappear from conscious memory. Different senses have different capacity for monitoring time and triggering memory. Human perception of time is determined by feelings, emotions and sensations. Computers time is very different. Computer time has well defined intervals of equal length. System behaviour can be endlessly recorded in relation to time without distinction between one instance and another. The recording itself may deteriorate, but if replicated it may remain available on the Internet forever. Generation after generation of data storage technology has improved significantly and by now memory seems to be infinite. Humans operate on a completely different rhythm to computers. This makes it more difficult for humans and computers to relate find computer scientists Quillinan [22] and van Splunter [18].

However, when technology mediates human collaboration 'timing' is critical in online processes. One of the assumptions of this study is that in online collaboration new kinds of witnessing, in which sharing of time and place is no longer necessary, are evolving. Where before 'place' seemed to be the beholder of trust, in online collaboration 'time' is the beholder of trust,concludes social entrepreneur and Free Software advocate Abraham. In several interviews this conclusion was supported. But where in small companies it is a genuine challenge to find the rhythm that is good for all, especially in the large scale distributed work in the outsourcing industry time is the ultimate tool for control. AnthropologistsUpadhya [27] and Ilavarasan [28], who both did extensive studies in the outsourcing industry in India, come to this conclusion [30][31].

In small companies rhythm in the orchestrating of workflow is crucial, argues Wilson [25]. Weekly online meetings with business partners, feedback to software patches within a day, response time to clients in a limited amount of hours has to be established like rule. For every task a specific medium is used: email, chat, Skype or phone. With different collaborators different rhythms are established. Wilson argues that because of these rhythms people manage to collaborate for over 4 years now while living in three different continents. Part of the rhythm is that, especially with the business partners when new plans are made or trouble is serious, people meet in real life. Smaller problems are usually solved in company hierarchies. Most important is keeping a good rapport, spending some time on jokes and keep writing the courtesy lines. Spending time on these 'useless' things makes a significant difference in the smoothness with which collaborations, according to Wilson, evolve. In this case organizing time in an efficient way benefits the workers greatly. The fact that they all keep to the rhythm is an expression of respect [25].

Very different is the time management in the outsourcing industry in India. In the last decade the Indian outsourcing industry developed the Global Service Delivery model within its IT industry in which Indian companies provide services 24-7 worldwide. Fundamental to the Global Service Delivery model is that local Indian workers adapt to the timezones of clients abroad. Shifts around the clock one can find in a variety of professions, but the outsourcing industry organizes its time more profound. Every single day, nearly every minute of every person all sorts of technological systems monitor their work. This 'low trust' environment affects the people who work in it and triggers an unintended dynamic of low performance as result, noticed Upadhya [27]. The lack of control, the boring work and especially the organization of the business and its systems, which register people and their deeds in a highly technological industrial manner, create contradictions and conflicts. There is no concept of 'personal' time for professionals involved. People work 10- 14 hours a day and are being monitored constantly. Many professionals start to miss the human touch in their activities. As a result, psychological stress related diseases have become a factor in India's healthcare as never been before, argues Ilavarasan [28].

Implications for Healthcare

Genuine witnessing is embedded in Wilson's company. People know each other, have met in real life and sustain their relationships over time by using technology. Time is core to their online collaboration: by keeping the rhythm, by creating consciously patterns of presence and absence. Time is the beholder of trust. When transposing this experience to cyber therapy for example, it is clear that sustaining relationships in real life is necessary for witnessing online to be genuine and effective in its intention. If not, processes of projection and attribution will trigger false witnessing in Oliver's terms. However, in specific cases anonymity may be beneficial especially when moral conviction is at stake [3]. Further research needs to focus on whether and how a clear rhythm in online collaboration between client and therapist can structure these processes of attribution and projection, which are part of any therapeutic process, in a beneficial way. Patterns of presence and absence seem to be a requirement for genuine witnessing to emerge.

When transposing the experience of the outsourcing industry in India to future healthcare systems which are more and more directed towards constant collecting and distribution of data of clients and their health, it is clear that 'monitoring' in it self is not beneficial for the human beings involved. It may generate lots of data that have the potential to lead to thorough advice and scientific results. However, a low trust approach creates low performance with ultimately stress and depression as a result. 'Monitoring' is apparently very different from witnessing in Oliver's terms. The question is whether it is the monitoring, or the log-files or how the log-files are used, is to be held responsible. It is clear that when people sense or know that they are being monitored while not being in control, this is detrimental for well-being. In the outsourcing industry hierarchy and production values undermine people's response-ability and address-ability. In addition, no privacy is granted because every minute is recorded and every exchange is kept. In such a context witnessing becomes an exception.

5.2 Place: Global Roots in Locality, Emotional Space and Visual Logic

Where architecture and thinking about architecture has a tradition of millennia, only in the last few years has research focused on the sense of place in virtual environments. For many centuries the physical environment defined people's distinct sense of place. The sense of place was deeply intertwined with the social structures. Place is still a strong beholder of trust. Simple conversations on the mobile phone regularly start with the question "Where are you?" Three aspects of the sense of place in the merging realities relevant to the design of future health systems surfaced in the interviews: (1) working global, living local, (2) impact of emotions, and (3) the sense of space.

The first issue concerns the 'working global, yet living local' effect of place. In the global business environment people remain rooted in their local environment. In the IT industry people talk about 'becoming global', referring to a meaning of the word 'global' that somehow includes moulding behaviour into a model, which everyone can understand regardless of where they are from. But in spite of 'getting global', Upadhya finds that it really matters where a person comes from [27]. In international projects people attribute many of the problems to communication gaps or cross-cultural differences. Instead of seeing themselves as working in a common culture, the digital culture or global technology culture, people see themselves as being located in these very distinct traditional cultures. To Upadhya this shows that people, even when they are working in cyberspace most of the time, are, in fact, rooted in their localities [27].

The second issue that surfaces when addressing place in relation to health, is the fact that emotions have a great impact on the experience of place. Social relations, architecture and the environment shape an individual when growing up, indicates Bawa [24]. When people are involved in conflict, and feelings of discomfort, anger and resentment determine how one is capable of relating to others, all sense of space disappears. Even a large house can offer no space in such a case. Conflicts influence experience of place. The Internet influences the sense of place as well. In Srinadar, in Kashmir, for example, the state shut down the Internet during war and this aggravated people intensely, Bawa found. Where the state treats Internet as a medium, for citizens it is actually a utility. It is above all a space, a window to the world that one really needs in times of hardship. By shutting down the Internet the government shut the citizens off from the rest of the world. The relation between place (land and space) and the online world, between the real and the virtual, is not dichotomous. It all flows into each other and emotions have a significant influence in this, argues Bawa [24].

Thirdly the 'sense' of place is of importance. The sense of place is very strong because it is fundamentally defined by how one interacts with a space, explains architect Jansma [19]. By participating in a physical space, touching it, engaging with it, the perception and vision of the built world changes. When designing physical environments the human body is always key to the design: vision, hearing, physical constraints of human size. The experience of one's body is crucial for the sense of place. Rhythm, timing, breathing, looking, smelling, temperature, tactility and moving with the body through the space are all elements that influence the sense of place.Having identity in a space and knowing where you are, makes people more relaxed. For Jansma the question whether space has acquired a new communicative capacity because of technology that makes it possible to send each other 'some space', where before we could only send some language or things, is irrelevant. Space has always been communication from the designer of the space to the user, on a non-language level. It is a very authentic communication channel, which doesn't have another truth behind it. A person, who witnesses the pattern in a building or an online environment, will not see the logic behind it but will experience the logic. How people relate to/sense such visual logic is highly personal. New technology is making it possible to create form or space and give it enough complexity to make it interesting. It has a logic and quality of its own, according to Jansma [19].

Implications for Health Care

For future healthcare environments the design of place, and the notion of knowing where one is, is crucial to having identity and feeling secure. Local physical environments influence the online sense of place, just as local physical environments are influenced by the online world to which one has access. Emotions change the sense of place and place triggers emotions as well. The design of place is more complex than a mere offering of functionality. It communicates a visual logic of values and complexities to which human beings are sensitive.

5.3 Relation: Communion, Use, Engagement, Performance and Global Communication Skills

Human beings are in relation with each other and with their environment through the dynamics in relation, performance and global communication skills. From the perspective of the actor, three dynamics in relation have been mentioned in the interviews with respect to orchestrating communication processes in merging realities. Sood, having worked extensively with Nokia for example, makes the following distinction [20]. In interactions with human beings and other natural and intelligent life forms the first of the dynamics in relation is communion. Communion offers the possibility of a shared meaning. Secondly human beings can be a user of things or an environment. A user is aware of the instrumentality of his or her actions with objects and systems with which he or she interacts. Thirdly, pointed out by Hazra, a human being can be engaged with an environment. Engagement refers to a granularity of involvement, to the intensity of sustained interaction [16].

Dynamics of relations have different characteristics in the variety of social structures human kind has developed. For many centuries people have lived in centred communities. Centeredness evolves from an awareness of physical being and behaviour. In centred communities people share place and practice and have immediate feedback on their work and witnessed presence in the community. Centeredness is a quality that makes human beings viable and gives them the wits to survive, as designer Panghaal formulates[17]. In centred communities people are in communion with each other and their environment. Awareness of the instrumentality, of ones actions within the community is part of the shared meaning that evolves from being in communion, as is engagement.

In merging realities in urban environments *engagement* is the primary means with which relations are defined. Through engagement a shared meaning with others may evolve. Being a user is also part of being engaged. In merging realities engagement becomes the source for authenticity. One can be as authentic on Facebook as if one has lived on the same piece of land for over 80 years, argues Hazra [16].

Levels of trust define rules of engagement. Establishing trust in a technology environment is not easy, finds Kaul [29]. Kaul trains professionals who work in the outsourcing industry and she finds that establishing trust requires the development of specific competences. Integrity, sharing (confidential) information in an honest fashion is a first requirement for establishing trust. Secondly it is important to show capability; to be on time, to deliver work on time, to be consistent. Thirdly it is important to be clear about intentions. Building reputation is a fourth requirement; one has to realize that trust travels between people; the relationship one builds with one person will generate trust when one learns to know a connected third person [29].

Several of the experts interviewed comment on the issue of manifesting identity in relation to being engaged in the online world. Especially in professional environments manifesting identity requires strategic attention. In small companies people stage identities towards clients, as it is good for business, but between colleagues a shared meaning is constantly negotiated because people trust each other and are dependent upon each other as well, finds Wilson [25].

In the open source community one of the drivers for contributing to the larger libraries of work is the fact that one earns reputation by performing convincingly. *Performance* is very much tied into the concept of showing capacity, but also reflects on a person's identity in the open source community, states Abraham [26]. Trust is organized in very transparent ways in these open source communities and the 'benevolent dictator' who runs such communities can be held responsible in the end, as Abraham formulates it [26]. The transparency of published and documented work is characteristic for the open source dynamic and facilitates people to perform.

In large production environments, as in the outsourcing industry, a specific kind of personal performance is staged because people have to mould into the Global Service Delivery model, concludes Upadhya in her extensive study on the IT industry in India [30]. Workers are witnessed and stage an identity to be witnessed with, yet the space in which they can take responsibility and be witness is very limited. This leads to a staging of professional identity that reflects an image, inspired by Silicon Valley models of how a software engineer should be. The staged identity deeply invades the self-reflection of people involved and as a result there is a great discrepancy between the actual practice and the self-image of the software engineers involved [27].

When manifesting identity and performing witnessed presence the relation with the self is at stake. Where before people could have different identities in different environments, in the merging realities the bandwidth for identity has diminished dramatically. Because of distributed networks and the infinite storage of data, the performance of different identities will inevitably clash. Spending lots of time online in a variety of networks for several years now, Abraham notices that as a result people end up deploying the lowest common denominator of their identity in environments where on- and offline worlds merge [26].

To be able to work in a global context people have to learn and adapt to cross cultural communication and learn '*global communication skills*', argues Kaul [29]. These skills mostly focus on behavioural skills: to show that one understands, (instead of just understanding it in ones own mind), to show confidence, to learn to present professionally, to be aware of body language, to develop verbal skills, to manage expectations, to make clear what one needs, what one expects and what one wants to do with ones team and with the global teams [29].

Global communication skills are designed to help people communicate across cultures, to help people to witness and be witnessed themselves. However, in the low trust environment of the outsourcing industry these behavioural skills do not seem to prevent the rupture between performance and inner witness. Narayanan, director of Sristhi School of Art, Design and Technoogy, having witnessed the development of Bangalore since the 1950's, strongly states that ultimately in the end humanness, being witness to each other and connecting with one's inner witness, is a personal choice to trust [32]. One has to stand by this choice to trust and accept the consequences. Failing is crucial when one wants to learn and make things. Guiding people through processes of failing, finding ways to deal with it and energizing people's motivation again, is what true leadership in collaboration is about according to Narayanan [32].

Implications for Health Care

For the design of future health environments notions of engagement and performance are distinct. Through being engaged shared meaning and new use evolve. Engagement is triggered by desire, motivation, fascination, perseverance, necessity and more. Granularity and intensity of involvement have to be addressed. Secondly the notion of performance requires attention. How much performance is beneficial for human beings and how do people detach their 'inner witness' from their potential to be witness and be witnessed? It is clear that trust in the variety of social structures has a significant impact on how people relate and can or cannot be witness to each other. In merging realities trust benefits from a clear understanding of subject positions, from a matching of online with offline experiences, from acquiring global communication skills. Finding the wits to survive and having the courage to trust and possibly fail, is in the end a personal choice.

5.4 Action: Inscribing Physical Presence, Online Transactions and Performance Online

The experts interviewed referred to action with respect to inscribing physical presence, online transaction and performance online. To better understand 'acting' in merging realities in relation to *physical presence*, first the situation in the Dutch Courts of Law is discussed. Proof of actions is part of finding the truth in Law. In actions, as well as traces of these actions, technology plays a significant role.

In Law the witness is a distinguished persona and in the merging realities the court is faced with new questions and dilemmas, explains judge and professor of constitutional law Van derVlies [33]. In Law a witness has to be sworn in and by this act words become deeds as well. Lying, when under oath, is considered to be a crime. Especially in Court where witnesses often have intense emotions about the crimes discussed, the judge has to disentangle emotions and facts. To this purpose, judges first make a common ground in the emotional realm. Sadness and anger have to first be recognized and accepted before the unfolding of facts can be addressed, as Van derVlies finds in her practice as judge [33]. For the Law technology creates a 'void' and therefore technological evidence cannot be accepted on face value: an expert opinion on the validity of the artefacts is needed for the judge to be able to understand their value in the process of establishing facts in the process of law. A trusted expert needs to report on the validity of evidence. Also witnesses have to be physically present in Court, either in the Court of Law at which the Judge resides, or (currently in experimental phase) using videoconferencing technology, in another Court of Law in which a Trusted Third Party (TTP), eg another judge, witnesses the testimony of the witness. The oath is taken in front of the TTP. So far, being witness in processes of Law involves being physically present in front of the Law [33].

In the online world an individual only exists because of *transactions online,* argues Abraham [26]. There are two types of transactions. There are machine records of transactions and there are mediated witnessed interactions (editing of pages, public postings, making links, 'I show I know you'). Digital witnessing contributes to the establishment of reputation and authenticity, through hyperlinks and records of transactions between humans and machines as well as between humans mediated through machines. One has to do transactions all the time to prove existence in time and space, finds Abraham [26]. As indicated in a number of previous sections, in the outsourcing industry recording of transactions is taken to the extreme. But also in a small company log showing that transactions have taken place proves physical presence at work. Log-files as well as the response time to each other's transactions online, are crucial indicators for people's presence and trustworthiness online [25] [27] [29]. Such transactions are part of production processes and are not geared towards a fundamental process as finding the truth and taking ethical responsibility in this process. Especially in the open source communities the transparency of transactions and the documentation of previous transactions while sharing work, creates a great sense of value, personal reputation and trustworthiness [25] [26] [27]. Apparently the dynamic of 'sharing' transactions is different to the one of 'controlling' transactions.

Testimony and presence in on- and offline environments is highly dependent on *performance*. Change in performance is another element that has been addressed in the interviews. Parthasarathi has studied the Indian music industry and has discovered the following phenomena [23]. In live performance of music the interaction between the singer and the listener is vital. The way the listener responds to what is being sung changes how the singer performs. In recorded versions of the same music the voice that could only be heard before at a special occasion is set free from the boundaries of time and place. As a result, the relation between the performer and the listener has changed profoundly: the context, the nature of the performance, the relation between the voice and the ear, the relationship between where the voice is coming from and where the voice is heard. The experience of listening to music has become anonymous for both the listener and the singer. If the singer does not know for whom he/she is singing then a more standardized composition will be the result, concludes Parthasarathi [23]. This resonates with the idea that in online environments people lose bandwidth for the performance of identity. Because relations are more anonymous, the nature of action is changed.

The primary quality of transaction between the real singer and the real listener is the physical relation of presence between them. The moment it is mediated there is not this real transaction but nevertheless people experience the mediated presence in the recorded music. In the mediated experience the cognitive understanding of what one is listening to, as well as the context in which one experiences the replayed music, mostly influence the experience, argues Parthasarathi [23]. Different media today create different kinds of presences dependent on how they facilitate different kinds of transaction in time and place. The telephone for example offers synchronous dialogues and therefore it is not replay, it is 'live' transaction. Because people use technology devices, they also adapt to them. When focusing on adaptation the question arises how far the design of technology can stretch the human capability to adapt. It s clear that there are physical thresholds of weight, size, sound level, clarity of the screens and so on. When focusing on social or psychological effects of media-use one may ask very different questions, according to Parthasarathi, like for example what happens to the understanding of the national news when one watches it alone, with a group or with three generations present [23].

Implications for Healthcare

For future healthcare applications these questions are very relevant. Physical presence is distinct yet human beings adapt to mediated presence, find ways to establish authenticity and reputation online and find ways to perform presence in online environments. However, the effect of these solutions reaches further than is visible at first sight because apparent 'handy' solutions deeply influence how people establish trust and find truth. Synchronous mediated communication and just in time exchanges of transactions seem to be crucial for establishing trust. Time is this sense, as stated before in section 3.3.1 is the beholder of trust. For future health applications in which online communication is vital, orchestrating a time design in transactions is distinct. The nature of transactions online in the interaction between the witness and the one who witnesses online, is determined by the limited possibility to perform one's presence. The context in which the mediated communication is perceivedhas great impact on how the communication is experienced.

5.5 Discussion of the Results of Exploring Witnessing in the Four Dimensions of the YUTPA Framework in Relation to Future Healthcare Issues

As computers are capable of many different types of interaction they have been attributed with many different qualities. In 1966 Weizenbaum's program Eliza showed that the endless patience of a computer posing repetitive questions modelled after Rogers conversational style of psychotherapy, convinced people to freely express their experiences and true feelings. The fact that the computer is there and like the stuffed animal or the doll does not get impatient and therefore freely allows for processes of projection and attribution, is part of the success of this program. Today when surfing anonymously on the Internet, and using that hole in time that is available 24/7, these processes of attribution and projection are at least as strong. In some cases these processes are effective, contributing positively to the health of people in, for example, anonymous help with abortion [34]. Digital interventions through low threshold self help programmes are proofed to be significantly successful in curbing drinking problems [35]. In other cases, as is the case with anorexia sites for instance, the processes of attribution and projection seem to confirm pathological behaviour and are destructive for many young women involved [3].

The question these developments pose is how much 'realness' people need to be able to be responsible for their own well-being and survival. When designing future health environments 'realness' can be the result of any one of the 4 dimensions of the YUTPA framework. Time design can offer synchronicity and just in time transactions. Place design has to respect the locality of the people involved. It may resonate or even trigger emotions and by its design will influence how people feel. Relations have to be established in the merging realities. Through being engaged in different kinds of presence, in physical presence and in the different media that are available, shared meaning may evolve. In the establishment of relations the confusion between systems and human mediated communication, between communion and use, may be profound. Over time people will realize the differences between types of systems and especially in crisis situations people will know in which systems or people to place their trust. Action in online environments is largely dependent on transactions. Through series of transactions the sense of interaction emerges. As in real life controlling transactions offers a very different dynamic than sharing transactions. Sharing work through transaction is beneficial for many people involved. The performance of presence in online environments does not support a rich enactment of identity and is dependent on the orchestration of series of transactions. For certain health environments anonymity and no physical presence is beneficial, yet synchronicity of transaction is vital.

Others need physical presence only once in while and will benefit for asynchronous transaction in between.

Future health environments need to take into account that:

(1) time is orchestrated to be the beholder of trust
(2) on- and offline place are designed to support emotional well-being with respect of the locality of the people involved
(3) the relationship between people has been established in an offline context, will enable health applications that support response- ability, address-ability, transparency of subject positions and the performance of testimony, contributing to the humanness of people involved. Mutual witnessing is the result. In specific cases anonymity may be beneficial for people involved. Further research has to show how witnessing in such cases can or cannot be orchestrated.
(4) Series of transactions online create a sense of interaction in which patterns of (physical) presence and absence are distinct.

6 Witnessed Presence and Systems Design

In merging realities systems transparency is leading in design. Users need to understand the roles they play in interaction with a system, and the responsibilities associated with these roles. The same holds for the systems with which users interact: their roles must be transparent as must be their responsibilities. Systems have the responsibility to manage interaction with users, their own processes, user data and system data responsibly. The subject position of both the user and the systems must be transparent. In this chapter the YUPTA framework has been used to analyse the elements that determine subject position.

With respect to Time this chapter argues that synchronisation of rhythm is core to trust. Systems and users need to synchronize their rhythms when presence in interaction is of importance. Systems and users also need to be designed to support different patterns of presence and absence in their own roles and in their interaction.

With respect to Place this chapter emphasizes the importance of experiencing place-ness and supporting well-being of human beings in system design. Visualisation plays an important role in this respect. Transparency of place-ness and well-being of data (ie location and integrity) is also a requirement for system design.

With respect to Action this chapter stresses the need for transparency in action and interaction: transparency of conduct between agents and human beings, transparency in the tasks and roles and responsibilities in their interaction, is essential to trust and integrity.

With respect to Relation this chapter identifies the need for transparency in the relations between the roles humans and systems play. The distinctions between human/human, human/system/, system/system, but also transparency with respect to their interaction with their environment, needs to be made explicit.

Transparency, integrity, identifiability/traceability, privacy, autonomy, and trust are key concepts identified by Brazier, Oskamp, Prins, Schellekens and Wijngaards for the design of actor-agent systems (systems in which autonomous software systems interact with human actors) from the perspective of legal acceptance [36] [37]. These concepts are very closely aligned to the concepts developed within the here presented study.

Designing systems to support the types of requirements identified above involves multiple challenges. Hardware, operating systems, middleware platforms and applications, and their interaction in different environments, together determine if and to which extent the above requirements can be fulfilled. Each computer system, for example, has its own rhythm, its own clock. The operating system translates information provided by the hardware to a concept of time. This notion of time is used by middleware platforms and applications to synchronise interaction with human users and other computer systems. The time experienced by a user in interaction (within a virtual environment for example), although abstracted from the underlying computer systems, is often not identical. Applications define how interaction with the human user, with other automated systems and with the environment is structured in the context of a social structure, relying on the functionality provided by the hardware, operating system, and middleware. Applications define how time is experienced. If, however, the underlying levels in system architecture fail, so will the time experienced. In the synchronisation of the clocks, participation and interaction between human beings and systems acquire meaning. Ultimately the applications define the rhythm in interaction, define absence and presence, in the experience of the user.

New types of systems in which multiple realities are involved, requires iterative processes of design to make such systems beneficial to human well-being. To this goal, 'realness' is a factor of distinction but only evolves in series of transaction and interactions between different systems. Orchestrating trajectories, using trade-off, making up for loss of YUTPA at certain moments by creating synchronicity of time or place or shared action in between, requires interaction with the clock.

Social structures define a human beings subject position. Many systems mirror existing social structures and the division of power within these structures. The Internet, however, has created the ability to create new social structures, creating new roles for human users. The creation of autonomous computer systems (both hardware and software) is creating new forms of agency both for technological agents and for human beings as well. New insights and skills are required for human beings to deploy these systems, taking responsibility for their own well being in the biological, social and technological realities as they merge.

7 Future Research

Soldiers can be taught to work together, to learn social skills and effective collaboration in specific situations in VR environments and many more [38]. But can a soldier who returns from war go to a VR environment and learn to deal with his trauma? Can the machine listen to his pain? Can a person who is not there but definitely listens by phone for example, help him out? Literally out of his trauma by offering to be witness and sharing responsibility for his testimony? Can we share responsibility in online environments? Situations and trauma that a war veteran faces, reach beyond individual destiny but demand political and social commitment as well [39]. Frantz Fanon already argued, that every individual change needs a social context to behold this change [40]. Can a networked systems environment offer such a social context?

How virtual environments and physical environments collaborate for the well-being of people involved is a new domain of research [41]. The here presented work shows that such research should have the ambition to move beyond cognitive behavioural therapy, in which virtual environments are used more and more already today. Health and well-being are more complex. Further research into witnessing will focus on how response-ability and address-ability and the locality of subject position can be shaped, when not sharing place. Time design will be in the focus of attention in this work.

Acknowledgement. The authors are grateful to StichtingNLnet for their support for this project, to Leen de Baat for filming and editing the interviews and to Thomas Quillinan for constructing the site http://www.systemsdesign.tbm.tudelft.nl/witness/ to host the information on which this chapter is based.

References

1. Kuhn, T.S.: The road since structure, philosophical essays, 1970–1993. In: Conant, J., Haugeland, J. (eds.) Autobiographical Interview, The University of Chicago Press, Chicago (2000)
2. Giddens, A.: The Constitution of Society, Outline of the Theory of Structuration. Polity Press, Cambridge (1984)
3. Caroline, N.: Presence and the Design of Trust. PhD diss., University of Amsterdam (2007)
4. Riva, G., Waterworth, J.A., Waterworth, E.L.: The Layers of Presence: A Bio–cultural Approach to Understanding Presence in Natural and Mediated Environments. Cyber Psychology & Behavior 4(7), 402–416 (2004)
5. Damasio, A.: Looking for Spinoza, Joy, Sorrow and the Feeling Brain. Vintage, Random House, London (2004)
6. Butler, J.: Bodies that Matter, on Discursive Limits of Sex. Routledge, New York (1993)
7. Caroline, N.: Witnessed presence and the YUTPA framework. PsychNology Journal 'Ethics in Presence and Social Presence Technology' 7(1) (2009), `http://www.psychnology.org`
8. Fukuyama, F.: Trust, Social Virtues and the Creation of Prosperity. Free Press Paperbacks, Simon & Schuster, New York (1995)
9. Peter, S., OttoScharmer, C., Jaworski, J., Flowers, B.S.: Presence, exploring profound change in people, organizations and society. Publsihed by arrangement with Society for Organizational Learning (2004), `http://www.solonline.org`

10. Kleiner, A.: Karen Stephenson's Quantum Theory of Trust. In: Strategy + Business, Fourth Quarter (2002), http://www.strategy-business.com (accessed 24 November, 2006) (retrieved)
11. Oliver, K.: Witnessing, beyond recognition. University of Minnesota Press, Mineapolis (2001)
12. IJsselsteijn, W.A.: Presence in Depth, PhDdiss., Technische Universiteit Eindhoven (2004)
13. Volkmer, I. (ed.): News in Public Memory, An International Study of Media Memories Across Generations. Peter Lang, New York (2006)
14. Foucault, M.: Parrèsia, Vrijmoedig spreken en waarheid. Trans. Ineke van der Burg. UitgeverijParresia, Amsterdam (2004); Original text Discourse and truth: The problematization of parresia, transcript of 6 lectures by Foucault at Berkeley, University of California (1983)
15. Practices, U.: Conference organized by Waag Society Amsterdam. The Virtual Knowledge Studio (KNAW) and the Arts and Genomics Centre of the Univeristy of Leiden (2009)
16. Hazra, A.: Witnessed Presence and Systems Engineering, Interviews by Caroline Nevejan (2008), http://www.systemsdesign.tbm.tudelft.nl/witness
17. Panghaal, J.: Witnessed Presence and Systems Engineering, Interviews by Caroline Nevejan (2008), http://www.systemsdesign.tbm.tudelft.nl/witness
18. van Splunter, S.: Witnessed Presence and Systems Engineering, Interviews by Caroline Nevejan (2009), http://www.systemsdesign.tbm.tudelft.nl/witness
19. Jansma, R.: Witnessed Presence and Systems Engineering, Interviews by Caroline Nevejan (2009), http://www.systemsdesign.tbm.tudelft.nl/witness
20. Sood, D.A.: Witnessed Presence and Systems Engineering, Interviews by Caroline Nevejan (2008), http://www.systemsdesign.tbm.tudelft.nl/witness
21. Warnier, M.: Witnessed Presence and Systems Engineering, Interviews by Caroline Nevejan (2009), http://www.systemsdesign.tbm.tudelft.nl/witness
22. Quillinan, T.: Witnessed Presence and Systems Engineering, Interviews by Caroline Nevejan (2009), http://www.systemsdesign.tbm.tudelft.nl/witness
23. Parthasarathi, V.: Witnessed Presence and Systems Engineering, Interviews by Caroline Nevejan (2008), http://www.systemsdesign.tbm.tudelft.nl/witness
24. Bawa, Z.: Witnessed Presence and Systems Engineering, Interviews by Caroline Nevejan (2008), http://www.systemsdesign.tbm.tudelft.nl/witness
25. Wilson, R.: Witnessed Presence and Systems Engineering, Interviews by Caroline Nevejan (2008), http://www.systemsdesign.tbm.tudelft.nl/witness
26. Abraham, S.: Witnessed Presence and Systems Engineering, Interviews by Caroline Nevejan (2008), http://www.systemsdesign.tbm.tudelft.nl/witness

27. Upadhya, C.: Witnessed Presence and Systems Engineering, Interviews by Caroline Nevejan (2008), http://www.systemsdesign.tbm.tudelft.nl/witness
28. Ilavarasan, V.: Witnessed Presence and Systems Engineering, Interviews by Caroline Nevejan (2008), http://www.systemsdesign.tbm.tudelft.nl/witness
29. Kaul, P.: Witnessed Presence and Systems Engineering, Interviews by Caroline Nevejan (2008), http://www.systemsdesign.tbm.tudelft.nl/witness
30. Upadhya, C.: Management of culture and Management through Culture in the Indian Outsourcing Industry. In: Upadhya, C., Vasavi, A.R. (eds.) An Outpost of the Global Economy, Work and Workers in India's Infrmation Technology Industry. Routledge, New Delhi (2008)
31. Ilavarasan, P.V.: Software Work in India: a Labour Process View. In: Upadhya, C., Vasavi, A.R. (eds.) An Outpost of the Global Economy, Work and Workers in India's Information Technology Industry. Routledge, New Delhi (2008)
32. Narayanan, G.: Witnessed Presence and Systems Engineering, Interviews by Caroline Nevejan (2008), http://www.systemsdesign.tbm.tudelft.nl/witness
33. van der Vlies, I.: Witnessed Presence and Systems Engineering, Interviews by Caroline Nevejan (2008), http://www.systemsdesign.tbm.tudelft.nl/witness
34. http://www.womenonwaves.nl
35. Riper, H.: Curbing Problem Drinking in the Digital Galaxy. PhD diss. Vrije Universiteit Amsterdam (2008)
36. Brazier, F.M.T., Oskamp, A., Prins, J.E.J., Schellekens, M.H.M., Wijngaards, N.J.E.: Anonymity and Software Agents: An Interdiscplinary Challenge. AI & Law 1-2(12), 137–157 (2004) ISSN 0924-8463
37. Brazier, F.M.T., Oskamp, A., Prins, J.E.J., Schellekens, M.H.M., Wijngaards, N.J.E.: Law-Abiding & Integrity on the Internet: a Case for Agents. AI & Law 12(1-2), 5–37 (2004)
38. Wiederhold, B.K.: The Potential for Virtual Reality to Improve Health Care. The Virtual Reality Medical Center (2006), http://www.vrphobia.eu (accessed at October 10, 2009)
39. Caruth, C.: History as false witness. In: Ekman, U., Tygstrup, F. (eds.) Witness Memory, Representation and the Media in Question. Museum Tusculanum Press, University of Copenhagen (2008)
40. Fanon, F.: Black Skin, White Masks. Transl. Charles Lam Markmann. Grove Press, New York (1967)
41. Riva, G.: From Virtual body to real body: virtual reality as embodied technology. Journal for Cyber Therapy and Rehabilitation 1(1) (Spring 2008)

Appendix

Interviews can be found at http://www.systemsdesign.tbm.tudelft.nl/witness. For convenience short descriptions of the interviewed persons are given below.

Sunil Abraham is director Policy of the Centre for Internet and Society is a Bangalore based social entrepreneur and Free Software advocate. He founded Mahiti in 1998, which employs more than 50 engineers today. Between June 2004 and June 2007, Abraham managed the International Open Source Network a project of United Nations Development Program's Asia-Pacific Development Information Program serving 42 countries in the Asia-Pacific region.

ZainabBawa works as an independent researcher on issues of urbanism, governance and impact of technology on political practices and institutions. Currently Bawa is pursuing her Ph.D. from the Centre for the Study of Culture and Society (CSCS) in Bangalore. In the past, Bawa has traveled extensively and has worked collaboratively with researchers in Kashmir and in Bangladesh on issues of space, conflict, violence and their impact on society.

AbhishekHazra is a visual artist based in Bangalore. His work explores the intersections between technology and culture through the narrative device of a 'visual fable'. He is interested in the social history of scientific practices, and his current, ongoing project attempts to explore the history of science research in colonial India. Hazra works with animated shorts and digital slideshows that often integrate textual fragments drawn from fictional scenarios. He is also interested in the way in which the languages of science journalism and information visualisation participate in the complex dynamics of 'knowledge dissemination' and 'translation'.

P. VigneswaraIlavarasan is presently Assistant Professor in the Department of Humanities and Social Sciences at Indian Institute of Technology Delhi. He obtained his PhD (Sociology) from the Indian Institute of Technology (IIT) Kanpur. In the last few years Dr. Ilavarasan did extensive research on the culture of the IT industry, India's booming sector since the mid 1990's.

Rein Jansma is architect of many public buildings and mobility throughout the Netherlands, Dubai, Georgia and more. Around 1990, together with Moshe Zwarts, Rein Jansma founded Zwarts&Jansma architects. They build soccer stadiums, railway stations, bridges, tunnels and other mobility infrastructure. In 1992 Zwarts&Jansma created the Dutch Pavilion on the world expo in Seville.

PriyaKaul is psychologist and a practicing therapist in Bangalore, India. She is consultant with CWSolution, a firm that facilitates workshops on leadership development, cross-cultural awareness and professional skills. Kaul has over 10 years experience with business development.

Geetha Narayanan has been at the forefront of the developing digital industry in Bangalore, India's renowned ICT centre for several decades now. Being the founder and director of the Srishti School of Art Design and Technology, she has been developing and implementing programs that blend design thinking, problem, project or place based learning with new digital technologies. Geetha Narayanan is formally trained in mathematics and international education. Currently she is finishing her dissertation "Complexity and System Thinking, Memetics, New Technologies, Learning and Social Change" at Sheffield Hallam University.

JogiPanghaal is concerned with the shift from product to service design, with a special focus on how craftsmanship and traditional artisan communities can be an inspiration for the design of services in current modern societies. For many years Panghaal was a contributor to Doors of Perception, a conference and network in which design, industry and social science collaborate to develop new ideas for service design. Panghaal graduated in Product Design from the National Institute of Design (NID) in Ahmedabad, India in 1977. Mr. Panghaal has been a visiting teacher at National Institute of Design in India, ID, at Les Ateliers Paris, at the School of Planning and Architecture, Delhi and at the GerritRietveld Academy in Amsterdam.

VibodhParthasarathi studies the music industry in the context of the Indian communication industry under globalisation, comparative media policy, and environmental movements & communication practices. His association with the media industry in India and abroad has varied from being a consultant, television producer and documentary director. He is one of the series editors of the Sage series on 'Communication Processes'. Currently Parthasarathi is reader at the Centre for Culture, Media and Governance at JamiaMilliaIslamia in Delhi.

Thomas Quillinan is a Security Researcher at the D-CIS Research Lab in Delft, in the Netherlands. He received a Ph.D., in the area of Security for Distributed Systems, and a M.Sc. in Computer Science from University College Cork in Ireland.

Dr. Aditya Dev Sood is the Founder and CEO of the Center for Knowledge Societies in Bangalore and Delhi, where he directs design and innovation projects involving peer-to-peer networks, interactive services and interface design, as well as product design. With foundational training in Architecture and Critical Theory from the University of Michigan, he is a former Fulbright Scholar with doctorates in Socio-Cultural Anthropology and Sanskrit Philology from the University of Chicago.

Sander van Splunter is a researcher at the Intelligent Interactive Distributed Systems (IIDS) (http://www.iids.org) at VU University Amsterdam, and at D-CIS lab in Delft. He has a background in Artificial Intelligence. His central research topic is autonomous adaptation of complex systems.

Carol Upadhya is associate professor at the National Institute of Advanced Studies in Bangalore. She has widely published and also made three ethnographic films 'Coding Culture: Bangalore's Software Industry' in collaboration with GautamSonti (NIAS-IDPAD project 2006). With A R Vasavi she edited the revealing study '"In an Outpost of the Global Economy: Work and Workers in India's Information Technology Industry" (New Delhi: Routledge, 2008).

Prof. Dr. I.C. (Inge) van derVlies is professor of Constitutional Law and Art and Law at the University of Amsterdam. She has served as part-time judge to the higher court in Amsterdam. She has widely published on a variety of perspectives on legislation, including international developmental perspectives. She is member of the Board of the European Association for Legislation and editor of the Dutch Judicial Journal. Van derVlies is a highly respected counselor and mediator in political and legislative issues. She chairs a variety of special commissions for local and national government agencies in the Netherlands. Van derVlies also worked as a counselor for the promotion of the rule in various countries like Indonesia, Ethiopia and former eastern European countries.

MartijnWarnier graduated with a Masters of Science in Cognitive Artificial Intelligence from Utrecht University, the Netherlands, in the beginning of 2002. He did his PhD in the Security of Systems group at the Radboud University in Nijmegen. His research focused on Language based Security and the mathematical formalization of properties such as non-interference, confidentiality and integrity. For the last three years he has worked as a Postdoctoral Researcher in the Intelligent Interactive Distributed Systems group at the VU University Amsterdam. Since September 2009 he is appointed the position of assistant professor at the TU Delft. His current research interests, besides security, include the interdisciplinary research field of Computer Science and (Computer) Law, and Self-organizing and Autonomic systems. In his free time MartijnWarnier loves acting in the theatre.

Rebekah Wilson obtained a degree in Composition at Victoria University of Wellington, New Zealand in 1996. Working as an independent composer, electronic musician, installation artist and filmmaker Rebekah Wilson has performed and lectured in many venues and festivals. Earlier this century she held the position of Artistic Co-Director at STEIM (Studio for Electronic and Instrumental Music), where she curated and participated in international festivals, workshops and education programs for live electronic and instrumental music, installations and film. Since 2004 she is the co-founder and director of technology for an international software development company, Source-Elements, delivering high-fidelity real-time audio delivery over IP. She is currently living between Barcelona and New Zealand and has taken up surfing.

Author Index

Made in United States
North Haven, CT
11 April 2023

35324749R00137